Revived!

Proven Natural Solutions for

Low Blood Pressure

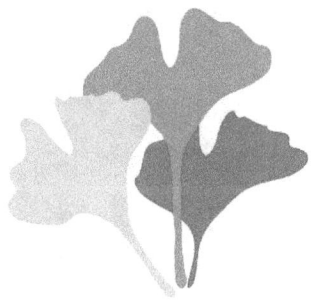

Dr. Dorothy Adamiak, ND

LiveUthing Press

ISBN-13: 978-1530975419
ISBN-10: 1530975417

Disclaimer

All information provided in this book is for educational purposes only. The information is not intended as a substitute for the medical advice of physicians. The reader should regularly consult a physician in matters relating to his/her health and particularly with respect to any symptoms that may require diagnosis or medical attention. This information is not intended to replace clinical judgment or guide individual patient care in any manner.

Use of this book implies your acceptance of this disclaimer.

To my husband, Andi,

For unconditional support,

Passion for self-improvement,

Thought provoking commentary,

And daring dreams that became reality

Table of Contents

Every book starts with a story....

For many years I had chronic fatigue. I was lifeless, depressed, and unproductive. My family doctor did all sorts of blood work, all of which turned out normal. I was pronounced "healthy." Meanwhile, I did not feel so. I could not hold a job, read a page without forgetting, and did not understand my woozy feeling in my head. I did not know why I felt worse after exercise and why exertion felt different to me than to other people. I worked diligently, but my efforts were not rewarded by expected results. Everything felt hard, difficult, and tedious. Because of that I learned to procrastinate. I was slowly turning into a sloth.

It was frustrating. My doctor said I was "well" and suggested I would benefit from talking to a psychotherapist or maybe go on an antidepressant. Otherwise, there was nothing wrong with me. Despite health assurances, my life continued on a slow and wearisome path, nothing I would call healthy.

I took my doctor's advice and consulted a psychotherapist that said the same thing as my family doctor: "there is nothing wrong with you." So what now? Whom do I go to? Who can help? I was completely disappointed with my diagnosis. Since getting help was futile I decided to take my health in my own hands.

Totally frustrated, one day I got a strange idea: I am going to become a doctor myself. Either I will find a cure or my life would continue being miserable till no end. So I did. I enrolled in university prerequisites and later in a four year accredited program to become a naturopathic physician. I was so determined that I finished with top marks and in 1999 got an official licensing number.

My continuous interest in chronic fatigue led me to look carefully at major health influencers: digestive, immune, and nervous system, as well as hormones and circulation. I was tireless and passionate about finding out the answers to chronic diseases and eventually I got rewarded. Over the years I managed to put the missing health pieces together for myself and my many patients.

Today, after gathering experience through two decades of clinical practice and sifting through a high-rise stack of research papers I know I can help you fast-track your own journey towards feeling your greatest.

So have a great read. Learn, discover, and get back to health.

DrD

Tools & Tests

Throughout the book you will come across **tests** and **tools** you may want to have. You will find them in our store grouped under the category "**book tools - revived**".

Alternatively you can click through to the category "**blood pressure**" to see what else your heart may need.

Our STORE: **LiveUthing.com**

DrD Blog: **DrDNaturopath.com**

Section 1

What's the fuss about?

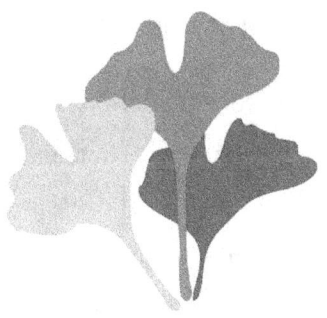

Chapter 1

Worse than high blood pressure?

Hypotension has never been a hot topic. There is not enough drama around it to raise eyebrows or cause a sense of urgency. Doctors *don't* see low blood pressure as a significant disease or an urgent concern. It is generally known that low blood pressure, in contrast to high blood pressure, does not pose a lethal danger. People don't die of *low* blood pressure. They die of *high* blood pressure.

It is *high*, not *low* blood pressure that is a dangerous killer, a source of strokes that is capable of permanently causing damage or even taking one's life within minutes. But low blood pressure is nothing like that. It is quiet, chronic, and frustrating. One can live with it for a long time. Due to the apparent mildness of the condition a standard prescription for low blood pressure is limited to "monitoring" rather than "medicating."

Not surprisingly just like health care providers, the sufferers themselves are also not sufficiently alerted to dangers of low numbers. Due to lack of alarming news in the media, an easy-going approach of doctors, slowness of progression of the condition, patients think of it more like an annoyance rather than a lethal disease.

However, behind a mild demeanor hides a sneaky health robber. This deceivingly mild condition, which nobody blames for any wrongdoing, turns out to be a total health nightmare. Just like a river capable of eroding shores and flattening rocks, low blood pressure can do extensive damage to the body over time. It can lower vital capacity, reduce organ function, and even make permanent changes to the brain. Low blood pressure is not an innocuous, leave-it-alone and forget-about state. It is a hidden health hazard few seem to pay attention to.

Chapter 2

Missing diagnosis

So you think there is something wrong with your body. You feel weak, spacey, and sort of drunk in the head. You suspected low blood pressure may have been causing the symptoms and shared these concerns with your doctor. To your surprise he insisted that your blood pressure was good. However, he was not really sure why you had other symptom, because all blood tests came back normal.

Many patients with low blood pressure experience the same frustration. They learn quickly that since there is nothing abnormal on the blood tests or x-rays their symptoms are not taken too seriously. Although relieved that the symptoms are not caused by a serious disease they are distressed by the lack of medical attention. Perfect blood work does not change the fact that the symptoms are real and they affect every aspect of their lives from memory to physical performance.

Motley of blood pressure symptoms

Low blood pressure symptoms may be very confusing, because they do not manifest the same in everyone. The symptoms play chameleon and disguise themselves as other conditions. Surprisingly, fatigue is not always present. Low blood pressure can appear as shortness of breath, headache, stiff neck, cough, indigestion, even forgetfulness and can be easily be mistaken for digestive, respiratory, immune, or musculoskeletal ailments.

The inconsistency of the symptoms is further complicated by age, gender, health status, and medication. For example, hypotension in a young woman may manifest as daily headaches, while in elderly it can be felt as debilitating fatigue. Since diagnosis of hypotension is frequently missing, it is not unusual that headaches are blamed for stress and fatigue for old age. Why does such an apparently easy to diagnose condition cause such a problem to our medical system? There is a reason for it and it has nothing to do with your doctor's competence.

It`s not hypotension unless

In good medicine things are never wishy washy. Either you have something or you don't. There is no in between. Either you have diabetes or you don't. Either you have osteoporosis or you don't. Things are definite and for a reason. It helps doctors make proper decisions.

Doctors cannot treat patients for non-existent conditions. It is reasonable to think that a doctor cannot treat for Alzheimer's if he can't find any, and cannot treat hearing loss if you hear well. Things are not any different with blood pressure. Before any treatment begins there has to be a diagnosis. But here is the trick. The current medical system recognizes only high or low blood pressure. There is nothing in between. Your doctor can treat you either for "hypertension" or "hypotension," but not for normal or normal-low blood pressure. If you fall in those latter, you are out of luck.

Low blood pressure underestimation

Low blood pressure is easy to miss. Even though it has a plethora of negative effects countless people continue to walk about with untreated hypotension risking falls, dementia, eyesight, and hearing loss.

This under-recognition is not on purpose. There are many reasons for it. Firstly, health care practitioners see low blood pressure as a lesser health burden then high blood pressure, so the focus is on detection and treatment of highs, not lows. Secondly, low blood pressure is frequently masked by a temporary pressure increase due to excitement while at the doctor's office, thus low blood pressure is seldom confirmed by clinicians during the physical exam time. Thirdly, there is not any simple and gentle pharmacological treatment for hypotension. The existing drug protocol for low blood pressure is reserved for more serious cases.

Improving odds for better health

Lack of diagnosis of hypotension does not equal to living free from symptoms. Given the factors above it is not unimaginable that many people live with blood pressure negatively affecting their mood, energy, and productivity. Some unfortunates may even be treated separately for depression, hearing loss, and dizziness and subject to ingesting numerous useless pills while the real cause of the problem remains hidden and is left untreated.

Chapter 3

Constant fluctuations

Blood pressure is never steady. It adjusts to circumstances constantly. It may be low when you are reading a romance novel, washing dishes, or sitting in the backyard, but it may climb sky high while you are watching an exciting movie, playing tennis, or quarreling with a spouse.

Since a doctor's visit can be nerve wracking, or at least is not on the list of the most banal experiences, your cardiovascular system will reflect it. As the heart pumps with extra excitement, heart rate goes up and blood pressure does the same. The effect is that your doctor registers normal blood pressure numbers in the office; meanwhile, you are stuck with low blood pressure anywhere else. This blood pressure variability is the reason why many low blood pressure cases get missed by health care practitioners.

In order for your doctor to diagnose low blood pressure and start a treatment, or at least connect the dots between your symptoms and your heart, he needs to see blood pressure numbers below the normal limits. If the numbers tested in his office are above low blood pressure mark you will walk out with a diagnosis of a "normal blood pressure" and "you must have something else." Do not be surprised that instead of asking you for blood pressure log your doctor may be sending you for physiotherapy, gastroscopy, or chest X-ray instead. Misunderstanding is common.

You can play the game of hide and seek for many years, take endless tests, treat wrong illnesses and continue suffering from the same problems unless you and your doctor are fully aware of the whereabouts of your blood pressure outside his office.

Periodic lows

There is one more reason why detecting low blood pressure is difficult. Not everyone will have steady low blood pressure throughout the day. Many people experience isolated episodes of hypotension precipitated by specific activities (such as standing up), prompted by specific environmental triggers (e.g. rainy weather), or just occurring at a specific times (e.g. before menstruation).

There isn't any universal blood pressure mold everyone fits into. Everyone's heart is different. That's why understanding your own blood pressure pattern is vital. Knowing the details can prevent the confusion whether you have or don't have hypotension-related symptoms and give you a clearer idea about the underlying causes of blood pressure changes.

When you are on meds

If you experience blood pressure lows, before going any further, you need to carefully evaluate where they come from. Make a clear distinction if these lows are naturally occurring fluctuations or fluctuations artificially induced by the meds you are taking. This distinction will help you take proper action. Medication induced lows in contrast to natural lows need adjustment to anti-hypertensive drugs, not a separate treatment.

If you see low numbers do not leave the matters alone regardless whether the lows are induced by medication or are your own. They have the same negative effects on the body.

Numerous patients who take blood pressure medication do it faithfully without any intermittent checks between doctor's visits. They believe that since they are treating high blood pressure, hypotension could not be a foreseeable possibility. Unfortunately, hypotension is a very common side effect in people who take medication for hypertension. This is when blind trust in diagnosis and lack of intermittent blood pressure checks can make the patients and doctors dumbfounded about the source of fatigue, headaches, and confusion. Make it easier on your doctor. Keep a log! Without a log you and your doctor may forever be puzzled why you're experiencing a never ending list of symptoms despite well-chosen prescription medications. If you found a lot of lows, but your doctor gave you a diagnosis of high blood pressure you need to bring your findings to his attention. He did not give you wrong medication. He just needs to adjust it better. Your doctor is not a psychic. A well-recorded blood pressure log may be the biggest breakthrough you both can have.

Chapter 4

So, what's normal?

Blood pressure is said to be ideal when at 120/80 mmHg. But that does not mean that a different number is bad. Normal blood pressure can vary significantly among individuals and even low numbers like 110/70 mmHg or high numbers like 130/84 mmHg should not cause a concern. Because of this variability blood pressure numbers are grouped into different categories. Current guidelines divide numbers into normal, low, and high ranges. The rules are straightforward and easy to understand. However, before you start comparing your numbers to the chart, keep one thing in mind: normal blood pressure not only varies between individuals but also fluctuates depending on circumstances.

When is it hypotension?

The guidelines are also clear on what constitutes low blood pressure. The numbers must fall below 90/60 mmHg before "hypotension" can be named. But in order to get a hypotension *diagnosis* it is not enough to see low numbers once. And even though you repeatedly see such numbers at home, your honest word will never be sufficient for a doctor. He needs to verify the numbers himself. After all a weak battery or a tube leak on your personal monitor can easily play tricks on the results. Your doctor has to see the numbers several times in his office to be concerned about low blood pressure as a condition.

Should it fluctuate?

Blood pressure fluctuates constantly. This is its normal feature. The heart always tries to adjust its beats to satisfy the body's needs. Let's say it tries, but not always succeeds. For example, a blood pressure spike is a healthy heart response to exercise, but in some people blood pressure may go down instead, causing breathlessness and exhaustion. I met people who didn't like exercising because they felt it sucked too much of their energy. But the reason for exhaustion was exactly the opposite of what they thought. It wasn't exercise at all, but their mal-firing heart that was causing the trouble.

The heart may also do something else: increase blood pressure when it is not needed. For example, peak it uncontrollably during an emotional stress. A fiery disagreement with a spouse should not cause hypertension, just a slight blood pressure increase at most. How are your numbers when you get angry, frustrated, and under pressure? Unless you check, you wouldn't know.

Don't expect your doctor to see these dips and spikes if he checks your blood pressure only in his office. Be prepared to question his verdict. If your doctor says your blood pressure is good but you see otherwise be persistent and suggest more detailed testing.

People make errors. Doctors make errors. Life is not still. Did you know that as many as 40% of people diagnosed by doctors as having normal blood pressure may actually have hypertension?[1] Why such discrepancy? Because blood pressure measured while sitting still does not reflect the heart dynamics while living.

So what's your blood pressure on a daily basis? Carry the cuff with you and test blood pressure at different occasions: while listening to music, reading a novel, while chatting in a coffee shop, or sitting in a park while kids are playing. With this method you can see how your blood pressure behaves under various circumstances like while relaxed, bored, and maybe also hungry, or tired. If something does not look right consult a health practitioner for an interpretation.

So what's normal?

Here is a snapshot of the ranges for normal, low, and high blood pressure. Remember that these numbers apply to measurements taken at a normal *relaxed* state which actually means *sitting still*. The numbers do not apply when readings are taken during physical exertion or various activities. Do not use this chart for blood pressure taken while exercising or opening your credit card statement.

Blood pressure reference chart

		Top number (systolic in mmHg)	Bottom number (diastolic in mmHg)
☹☹	High blood pressure - extreme	Above 180	Above 110
☹	High blood pressure – stage 2	160 - 179	100 - 109
☹	**High** blood pressure – stage 1	140-159	90 - 99
😐	Normal high (pre-hypertension)	139 - 121	81 - 89
☺	**Standard - normal**	120	80
😐	Normal low	119 - 91	79 - 61
☹	**Low** blood pressure	Below 90	Below 60
☹☹	Low blood pressure – faint range	Below 60	

Section 2

Unsuspected Effects

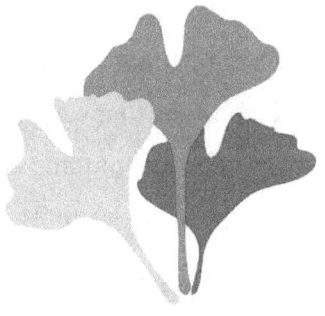

Chapter 5

Low isn't so safe any more

The innocence of hypotension is now coming into question. Low blood pressure has been shown capable of eroding health. Studies pointed out that although hypotension is not as deadly as hypertension, it does have a substantial long-term adverse impact on our well-being. Low blood pressure contributes to poor circulation. Cold hands and feet are common examples of this phenomenon. Low blood pressure also reduces oxygenation. Red blood cells that carry oxygen do not sufficiently reach vital organs if heart pumping is too weak. A brain that is in short supply of oxygen will feel foggy, dull and slow.

Poor circulation and poor oxygenation have a much more profound effect on our lives than previously thought. Hypotension can negatively affect brain function, mood, kidneys, coordination, and even life span. Even minute falls in blood pressure, falls that most doctors would dismiss as normal, have been found to have cumulative negative consequences.

Here are unsuspected effects of insufficient brain oxygenation:

- **Sensory impoverishment**: reduction in hearing and eyesight; this may manifest as bumping into things, tripping and falling, being prone to accidents; not hearing warning noises e.g. approaching car, sirens, and screams
- **Shift in demeanor**: personality changes, increasing anxiety, anger, and poorer interpersonal relationships; this may manifest as quarrelsome, inflammatory, conflictual personality
- **Loss of coordination**: difficulty with balance and movement; this may manifest as banging into things, slamming, hitting or dropping items
- **Visual impairment**: blurry vision, tunnel vision; this may manifest as difficulty reading signs, computer screens or newspapers
- **Communication issues**: slurring of speech, mispronunciation, difficulty forming sentences; this may manifest as dislike for participating in conversations and expressing self
- **Confusion**: exhibiting poor judgment, making wrong decisions; this may manifest as carelessness e.g. spending money unwisely or taking wrong turns while driving
- **Impairment of comprehension**: memory loss, forgetfulness; this may manifest as inattention e.g. missing a doctor's appointment or misplacing things
- **Bodily symptoms**: headaches, stiff neck etc; this may manifest as experiencing puzzling symptoms without any perceived cause

Your body symptoms may be your main clue that your blood pressure is changing. Be keen on detecting them, because your doctor's eyes may be looking only for high blood pressure effects.

Hypotension reduces life success

From lower grades on math exams, to slower reaction times while driving, insufficient brain oxygenation can affect many aspects of your life. Blood pressure decides whether you will have difficulty answering a question when confronted by a boss or can explain yourself when challenged by a family member. But low blood pressure would not only impair your perception and cognition, it can also affect the mood.

People with low blood pressure are found to have reduced motivation, increased feeling of hopelessness, and are less likely to put in any effort.[2] The resulting anxiety, depression and bad mood have far-reaching consequences at work and at home. They lead to unhappy interpersonal relationships, loss of satisfaction, higher stress, and lower productivity.

Depression, dementia, glaucoma, and life span

All body organs require good blood flow to function well. Low blood pressure makes things harder. Liver, kidneys, intestines, or muscles just can't work well if there is insufficient oxygen. For example, reduced blood flow to the liver can lead to slower digestion and detoxification as well as poorer blood flow to muscles can lead to a meager performance at the gym. It is not difficult to figure out that low blood pressure can make one toxic, bloated, and weak.

Studies point out that hypotension, in fact, does increase risk for developing specific health problems. Among them are:

- Increased chances for **depression** and **anxiety**. A very large 2007 study done on over 60 thousand subjects found that regardless of age people with chronic low blood pressure are significantly more prone to depression and anxiety[3]

- Increased risk for **dementia**. Difficulty thinking, memorizing, and impaired cognition is a well-known short-term effect of blood pressure drop, but a recent study involving close to one thousand participant pointed out that long term insufficient blood perfusion is found along *permanent* changes to the brain. Even arrhythmia (skipping beats) which results in temporary minor lowering of blood pressure can cause deep changes in white matter of the brain.[4]

- Increased risk for **glaucoma**. A small study correlated reduction of visual field with excessively low blood pressure at night. The study found that the depth and the duration of blood pressure dips at night correlate strongly with the severity of vision loss. This visual impairment happens regardless whether the dips occur spontaneously or are induced by medication.[5]

- Decrease in **hearing** acuity. As per a research done at University of Bologna, Italy, hypotension can be blamed for hearing loss even in younger individuals. This 1999 study found that people with numbers below 105/60 mmHg have more than twice the risk for hearing impairment than people with higher numbers.[6]

- Onset of ear noises, **ringing in ears**, and vertigo.[7, 8]

- Increased risk for **kidney failure**. Recent studies show that acute kidney failure is typically preceded by an episode of low blood pressure.[9]
- Increased mortality in **infants** as well as their delayed motor development and hearing loss.[10]
- Shortened **life span**. An older 1989 study demonstrated that not only high blood pressure, but also "the innocent" low blood pressure correlates with a shortened life-span.[11]

Slower beats, longer life?

While researching heart function and longevity I have found another interesting correlation. This one does not directly involve blood pressure, but rather heart rate. Don't be overly preoccupied by the findings, though. Treat them more like fun facts rather than predictions written in stone.

A paper written by June Liu and published in *Undergraduate Journal of Mathematical Modelling* in 2011 found a significant inverse relationship between human longevity and heart rate.[12] According to this model people with slower heart rates live longer lives.

The study correlated an average resting heart rate of 70 beats per minute with an average life expectancy of 70 years. Faster heart rate correlated with shorter lives and slower beats with longer lives. As per the calculations, people with resting heart rate of 90 per minute should expect to reach a statistical lifespan of only 55 years. People with resting heart rate of 60 should enjoy an average of 82 years and people with 40 beats per minute can celebrate a fantastic 123 years.

Before grabbing your wrist to find the pulse be aware that this statistic may apply only to naturally occurring heart rate. Use of medication may invalidate data.

If your heart rate is a bit on a high side, don't panic. Find a way of reducing it, either by learning how to cope with stress better or by spending more time on cardiovascular conditioning. Regardless of whether you believe these numbers or not, investing in emotional and physical fitness is always a good idea. Emotional and physical strengths are top life assets. They will surely help with longevity regardless of your current pulse speed.

Chapter 6

Hypotensive personality

Do you know your personality type? Are you outgoing, reserved, task or people-oriented? Are you a thinker, a leader, a planner or a protector? You may be any of these, but if you have low blood pressure you also have a hypotensive personality.

Let's see if this may be true. Do you feel that low blood pressure causes foggy brain? Do you believe it lowers your ability to comprehend, memorize, and think? Are you worrying that your school grades or work productivity suffer because of diminished capacity? Do people think you are lazy or frail, because you dislike exercise?

Feeling tired, acting placid, and demure is normal for people whose lives have been touched by hypotension. But a transformation from a "life failure" to a life success may be just as easy as improving circulation. When blood pressure normalizes many "losers" and "wimps" magically turn into intelligent, smart, and gutsy folks.

Personality makeover!

Let's uncover the typical traits of hypotensive personality. See if you can recognize yours or someone else's qualities in the list below.

- **Apparent dullness**: Slow thinking, difficulty in understanding reading material, dullness that may be perceived as confusion or lack of comprehension
- **Unsteadiness**: Feeling of spaciness, whooziness, lightheadedness that reduces physical confidence and prevents experiencing full physical potential
- **Mental weakness**: Difficulty learning, trouble with focus and concentration; kids may have poor grades and dislike school
- **Anxieties**: Lack of zest for life, fearfulness, lack of confidence, sadness and depression; lack of motivation and general dissatisfaction with life for no discernible reason
- **Physical weakness**: Fatigue, dislike for exertion, apparent laziness, slow reactions that keep many from enjoying the more adventurous side of life
- **Frequent headaches**: headaches that are non-throbbing, but dull, pressing; that are bothersome, but not bad enough to seek medical attention
- **Weird sensations in the head**: Ear pressure and fullness, humming in ears that is annoying but seldom diagnosed as problematic
- **Excessively delicate nature**: Paleness and loss of musculature, frailness, loss of vitality and poor blood flow

- **Symptoms of poor circulation**: Cold hands and feet, sensitivity to cold; fungal infections on toes as fungus thrives in areas with poor circulation
- **Aesthetic difficulties**: Poor quality hair, hair loss, hair dullness that can frustrate to no end; fragile nails

Wow! Isn't it weird and somehow relieving to find out that what's painfully "stuck on you" is actually an expression of a cardiovascular imperfection rather than inherent personality traits? Genetic features are difficult to change, but traits developed due to poor circulation can be modified. There is no point chasing supplements for anxiety, avoiding physical intensity, or hiding from the windy outdoors if one can cure it all with better circulation. Depressive tendencies, physical frailness, or weak mental performance can improve together with blood pressure numbers.

Chapter 7

Do you dip well?

Don't get ready for dinner yet! This chapter won't tell you how to dip chicken wings in BBQ sauce or fries in ketchup, but whether your blood pressure behaves well at night.

Blood pressure, despite popular belief, does not stay steady throughout the day. Instead, blood pressure follows a nature-driven twenty-four hour cycle. Circulatory system has its own rhythm and diurnal fluctuations. Basically, it drives blood pressure up during the day and keeps it low at night. These rhythmic fluctuations attracted scientists' attention, who tried to establish whether different patterns correlate in any way with different levels of health. And if fact, discoveries were made.

Blood pressure in healthy people behaves differently at night than in those with poor health. In healthy people blood pressure goes down just a tiny bit, about 10-20%.[13] Anything higher and anything lower were correlated with various health problems.

But why would lower blood pressure at night be good? Night is the time for rest and even the never-stopping heart needs it. Small dips are a welcome sign of good health, a sign that relaxation occurs, and a sign that the process is fully controlled by the body. Larger dips or lack of them suggest that the nervous system and the heart are out of sync, not a healthy situation.

Things must go down overnight

So a small dip overnight correlate with better health, but what if there is no dipping at all? Would no change in blood pressure during sleep mean anything? Would it correlate with poorer health? Observations were very surprising and clearly suggesting that lack of overnight dips can be a warning sign for various health problems.

Studies correlated lack of blood pressure dipping with poorer sleep, night waking, and sleep apnea.[14] Non-dipping was also associated with enhanced risk of cardiovascular events[15] such as strokes and heart attacks as well as endocrine and nervous system dysfunctions[16] including hyperthyroid and various neuropathies. Non-dippers were found to be experiencing more stress, and have stronger family history of hypertension.[17]

Just like lack of dipping at night reverse dipping, or higher blood pressure at night were also related to health problems. But higher blood pressure at night, called nocturnal hypertension, was found to be even worse than a lack of dipping. Increased blood pressure at night was found to be present in a large proportion of people that had suffered a stroke.[18] Because of this finding many studies suggested that rise of blood pressure overnight should be taken seriously as a warning sign of a seriously compromised cardiovascular system. Some researchers proposed that when there is an increase in systolic (top) number one should take serious precaution. A major cardiovascular event may be near.[19]

Dipping extreme

If night-time dipping is good for a person with normal blood pressure, would the same be true for a person who has low blood pressure? Would that extra blood pressure dip at night cause problems in the morning?

I am sure you had mornings that felt as if your body could wake up despite sleeping sound all night. We all had mornings that felt blah. If they happened once in a blue moon, disregard it. However, if most of your mornings feel this way it's wise to check what your heart is doing at night.

Chronically tired mornings are definitely a concern. They aren't in any way correlated with good health. Although reasons for morning fatigue may be many, one of them is low oxygenation. Low oxygenation is directly related to exaggerated blood pressure dips at night and there are many extra dippers among us.

Extra dipping at night is never good, and especially troublesome for someone with low blood pressure. Extra-dipping means that blood pressure goes beyond the healthy drop of 10-20%.[20, 21] In extreme situations extra-dippers can go as low as 50 points below their daytime baseline, which is definitely too extreme for health. Extreme lows can, just as the extreme highs, lead to cardiovascular events and brain damage.[22] In extreme dippers the harm is due to insufficient blood flow to the heart and the brain. Exactly because of diminished of blood flow, people with extra-large dips are more likely to suffer silent strokes.[23] The extremes are not good for the eyes either, as lack of oxygen causes damage to the nerves and can lead to vision loss.[24]

Who do you think are those extreme dippers? Diabetics, people with hardened arteries[25] people with sleep apnea.[26] Extreme dipping and lack of oxygen may explain why diabetics are chronically tired, prone to nerve damage, and have higher incidence of vision loss.

Dipping after meals

Have you ever felt like having a nap after a meal? Interestingly, this is when your blood pressure fell and your brain was short of oxygen. Studies showed that close to 70% of the elderly in hospitals nap due to a significant blood pressure drop (at least 20 mmHg systolic) after every single meal.[27] It is not because sleeping pills slipped into potatoes by mistake, but because of circulatory and autonomic nervous system defects. Don't ignore post-meal naps. They are not a sign of good health.

How can you tell what your blood pressure is doing without obsessively squeezing your arm every minute or waking up in the middle of the night? There is a way. Ask your doctor to get you a Holter monitor, an automatic blood pressure reader. You will need to wear it for two days to get conclusive results, but you won't need to do very much. The Holter monitor will automatically check your blood pressure every few minutes and report the results to your doctor.

*You can find Holter monitor in our **LiveUthing.com** store*

Chapter 8

Secrets of a zestful morning

Blood pressure is one of the simplest things to check yet nine out of ten people do not know their blood pressure numbers.[28] Half of people with *high* blood pressure are unaware of it[29] and barely anyone with low blood pressure knows about their condition. And that's not because of lack of care.

Low blood pressure can easily get obscured because of natural blood pressure fluctuations. Many individuals experience dips of blood pressure intermittently throughout the day without having a clue about it.

I bet you don`t roll out your blood pressure monitor when your eyes open in the morning and test your blood pressure before putting your feet on the ground. Very few people do. Obsessive testing in the morning is generally not a popular activity. Morning is a time of rush, not leisure, and can get really hectic if one has to go to work. For most of us morning routines are efficiently shrunk to only essential procedures, which are usually devoid of optional health checks. It is safe to say that regardless of life arrangements there is a slim chance that blood pressure gets tested at dawn.

Tired, groggy, and dopy?

Some dopy, lightheaded, and dazed mornings may be nothing else but a sign of hypotension. But how would you ever guess that unless you get the monitor out right then and there to confirm the numbers? It is tempting to blame the morning fatigue on a "restless" night, but don't! Lazy mornings can be your best friend in exposing hormones in need.

Morning awake

What comes down must go up. And so is the case with the blood pressure. Overnight dips should be followed by day-time rises. The first noticeable peak is expected soon after waking. The body needs it to face the day and to transform the day from groggy to zestful. If the surge does not happen the morning will lack energy and zip. The "get up" of blood pressure reflects hormonal changes inside the body. The awake phenomenon follows a cortisol peak. Those who can`t wake up in the morning may be exactly the ones whose hormones need some TLC.

Cortisol, a powerful hormone, just like blood pressure, obeys a twenty-four hour cycle. Cortisol is expected to fall overnight and rise in the morning. Body alacrity depends on cortisol. Studies confirmed that morning release of this hormone is invariably followed by heightened alertness.[30] How much cortisol is released makes a difference. A higher cortisol peak leads to an easy wake up, good morning energy, and higher blood pressure. In contrast, low or a complete lack of cortisol, may not only result in low blood pressure, but also in fatigue and pain. That's because cortisol increases blood sugar and provides anti-inflammatory/anti-discomfort effect.

Here are some other cortisol facts in case you are curious:

- Highest cortisol peak appears just before waking
- Second cortisol surge can appear about twenty minutes after waking
- Three quarters of people are known to peak twice
- Cortisol-awake phenomenon is present in 77% of normal individuals.[31]
- The lowest cortisol point occurs during the deepest part of the night, around 3 a.m.
- Cortisol release can change when health is compromised

A healthy cardiovascular system welcomes a moderate blood pressure surge in the morning. It helps flood the organs with fresh blood and deliver sufficient oxygen to face the day. But, as life wisdom teaches us: all has to be in moderation. Surges above 140/90 mmHg should not be cheered for.[32] Low blood pressure during the day with a high spike in the morning is a cause for a real concern.

Cortisol flats

If you suspect cortisol flats you need to have a good look at your adrenals. These two little glands sitting on top of kidneys are largely responsible for cortisol production. If hormonal output is lagging, maybe it`s time to check the factory. It may be malfunctioning.

Malfunctioning adrenals are bad at their job. They do not produce sufficient cortisol for morning arousal. Suspect weak adrenals when you are unable to cope with stress, or when you feel nervous, anxious and apprehensive without a reason. Fatigued adrenals are not rare. They are common and they are known to turn a healthy, zestful, energetic morning into a lifeless, dull, and comatose drudgery.

But do not mistake adrenal fatigue with Addison's disease. These two cause constant confusion and misunderstanding between health professionals. Be aware that a conventionally trained physician will not be familiar with the concept of adrenal fatigue. He will only know Addison's disease. Asking your endocrinologist to diagnose adrenal fatigue will be futile. He cannot do it.

Addison's disease, which is the result of a complete exhaustion of adrenals, is relatively rare. It happens only in 1 in 20,000 people.[33] Addison's disease is easy to diagnose. A simple blood test will suffice and your MD can`t miss it.

A minor adrenal fatigue can affect blood pressure and lower energy, but a full-blown Addison's disease will be much more burdensome. Sudden body pains, low blood sugar, lethargy, or dark patches on the skin can show up only in major adrenal crisis, not in a minor glandular glitch. By the time one has Addison`s disease it is obvious to everyone.

Addison's disease is an extreme far end of adrenal fatigue and one may wonder how unlucky some people may be. But lack of luck has nothing to do with it. In the vast majority of cases adrenals do not go from healthy to exhausted overnight. It takes them years to reach that final stage. In the meantime they go through various phases. They start sluggish, then go weaker, and eventually their output fades away completely. Unfortunately there aren't any special medical tests to detect semi-failed adrenals and one cannot just draw blood for that. Despite diagnostic difficulties adrenal fatigue can still be pinpointed. This task can be accomplished with saliva samples.

To test for adrenal fatigue four saliva samples are collected over several hours. Once collected and labelled they will be sent to a specialized lab for analysis. The lab will be able to establish whether cortisol amount in the saliva follows a healthy curve. If cortisol is low in any of the samples adrenal fatigue is suspected and correct treatment is suggested. Many people with chronic fatigue are unaware that this test may be nothing short of "God-sent". It may provide a solid answer to why they feel lifeless, tired, unmotivated, and why blood pressure keeps below vibrant.

To have the test done look for a reputable laboratory and after you get results refrain from showing them to random health practitioners. Not everyone understands the results, so make sure you get someone who does. Your safest bet is to seek out a board-certified/licensed naturopathic physician or a medical doctor trained in functional medicine. These health professionals are familiar with various adrenal patterns including fatigue, burnout, exhaustion, and Addison's disease. Your family doctor may not be.

PS. You can find adrenal tests in our LiveUthing.com store

Chapter 9

What's with the morning sniffles?

Do you have a case of morning sniffles? You may think it's from allergies, but the sniffles can be actually a little-known side effect of night-time hypotension. There is no denying that anxiety, ear and eye problem, kidney malfunction, memory lapses are related to lower blood flow, but can a runny nose fit in that equation? There haven't been gobs of studies on the subject, but my clinical experience indicates that grogginess sniffles, body chills, and throat soreness can be common aftermaths of a hypotensive night.

These strange morning sniffles do not usually extend to the later part of the day. The "colds" and "allergies" disappear shortly after breakfast and seldom develop into a full-blown infection. Because the symptoms are transient and resolve quickly without lingering, the sniffling phenomenon is seldom mentioned to anyone. It becomes a "normal" feature of most mornings and one learns to "live with it."

Beyond the obvious

Nothing in the body happens by chance, not even a sneeze, thus recurrent symptoms need extra attention. Sniffles that do not want to go away are not any different than a scrape that does not want to heal. There is no point of gluing a different color band aid on the scratch. It won't change the outcome. If the scrape does not want to go away there must be a reason for it. Maybe the immune system cannot handle the wound or the blood flow is insufficient. Regardless of which one is true, it is safe to say that trying a different color band aid won't make it better. For the same reason if water keeps on dripping from the nose it would only make sense to look beyond standard nasal sprays and Kleenex tissues.

Hypotension and weak immune system go together. Low blood pressure means poorer circulation, and that means colder body temperature. Notice that people with low blood pressure get colder more easily. But poor circulation is not just about cold hands and feet. Poor circulation has further ramifications. A chilled body invites viruses.

The land of rhinovirus

A common nose virus called rhinovirus is a cold climate lover. You won't entice it with a beach chair, slippers, and sunglasses. No. It prefers a chillier environment. Healthy noses aren't cold enough. Rhinovirus won`t make a party there. The virus feels its best around 33-35°C (91-95 °F), which is 1-2 degrees Celsius below normal. At this temperature rhinovirus gets very amorous and makes lots of babies. In medical language we call it increased viral load. When viral load gets too heavy symptoms of cold or sniffles occur.

Interestingly the core temperature changes throughout the day. It fluctuates with activity. It keeps its lowest at night or morning, the time when we move the least.[34] This explains why sniffles, which are cold dependent, subside by mid-day, when the body warms up.

Healthy blood pressure can keep core temperature normal despite open bedroom windows and thin blankets. Low blood pressure doesn`t. A runny nose may be your first unusual indicator of poor circulation.

Does it mean that all morning sniffles come from hypotension? Absolutely not! How can anyone then tell whether the sniffles are from allergies or from low body temperature? Easy! Pull out a thermometer and test yourself.

BBT test

The test to measure morning core temperature is called BBT. BBT stands for "Basal Body Temperature". It is a test that measures metabolic fire. BBT may not only be helpful in detecting immune system flaws, but also in finding a hidden reason for stubborn weight. Low BBT indicates slow metabolism and this means weight loss isn't possible without serious calorie cuts.

BBT is tested first thing in the morning. Stay in bed and ensure that a working thermometer is within your reach (remember to put it on your side table the night before). Do not wonder off anywhere after waking.

Keep under cover, forget the bathroom, and leave your itch alone. Stay still. Slowly reach for your thermometer and start testing. Keep in bed and relax. Wait until the measurement is done and then check the temperature.

Normal oral temperature should be around 36.6°C (97.9°F). Temperatures below 36.3°C (97.3°F) may be the reason why the virus parties heavily in your nose. Do not be shocked if you see 35.5°C (95.9°F) or even 34.5°C (94.1°F) on your thermometer. "Arctic" body temperatures *are* common in low metabolic and low immune system states.

The dreaded trio

Have you just discovered that besides low blood pressure and morning sniffles you also have low BBT? This dreaded trio needs a special treatment as poor circulation has to be addressed first before the nose stops dripping. Don't spend endless money on Dristans, Sudafeds or other popular nose-drying sprays. You will only throw your money away in exchange for a few hours of relief. Instead think for a moment. If your "morning allergies" are due to low immune system, low temperature, and poor blood flow does it make any sense to use nose-drying sprays? They don't boost immunity, neither increase temperature, nor contribute to better circulation. Health is a skill, not a pill, potion, injection, or a cream. And for sure health does not come conveniently packed as a nose spray. There is always a reason why symptoms persist. Always look for underlying causes so you don't become a slave to varied-color band-aids.

Chapter 10

A dangerous act of peeing

If you think that falls happen only during the day and lying in bed is the safest time you are far from the truth. It is exactly the night that presents unexpected health risks. A combination of a finicky bladder and unpredictable whereabouts of your blood pressure may be a sure prescription for nighttime disaster.

Have you heard of people fainting in the bathroom? These are not old wives' tales. Bathroom fainting is a well-documented fact. And it is not as uncommon as you may think. About one in ten people faint at least once in their lifetime during urination.[35] But why people stumble at the toilet is no longer a mystery. We don't have to blame thick bathroom darkness and non-existing soap on the floor for falls any longer. Science has a much better explanation.

Did you know that peeing causes a drop in blood pressure? This is not due to loss of bladder pressure, but because of a neuro-cardiovascular feedback from voiding. Little things add up. When one combines night-time dipping with the pressure lowering effect of relieving the bladder, fainting becomes a real possibility.

Fainting numbers

Fainting does not happen with any random blood pressure drop. Blood pressure has to reach below 60 mmHg[36] before loss of consciousness occurs. But 60 mmHg does not pertain to the bottom (diastolic) number. Although hard to believe, this number refers to the top (systolic) reading. The body is exceptionally adaptable and can handle incredible adversities. When your blood pressure monitor reads 100/50 mmHg you may feel lifeless, but the numbers still have some descending to do before you would kiss the floor.

Fainting due to night urgency happens, not surprisingly, to older individuals as age makes both blood pressure and bladder control less predictable. Night fainting is more common in males for one simple reason: their urination-assisting projectile members operate best on standing.

If you ever made a night-time pee trip and somehow managed to see stars in a windowless bathroom you should find the next page interesting and possibly life-saving. Thirty per cent of falls end up with cuts and bruises. Twelve per cent end up with a broken bone.[37]

Prevention is the key

Accidents are accidents. They are never preplanned, so it is best to take precautions. Although stopping the bladder from waking you up may not be an option there are a few things you can do to avoid ending up flat on the floor:

- **Drink water**. That may sound counterintuitive, but there is wisdom in it. Water prevents dehydration, which contributes to low blood pressure. However, drink water during the day to prevent urgency at night.
- **Avoid alcohol.** Say no to that shot of whiskey at night. Alcohol is dehydrating and promotes urination. Goodnight drinks can lower blood pressure and increase bladder pressure.
- **Eat.** Do not go to bed hungry. Eat something before retiring. Low blood sugar can contribute to low blood pressure.
- **Use salt.** Do not be afraid of salt. It can keep your blood pressure higher.
- **Engage your MD**. Ask your doctor to switch the timing of your blood pressure medication (if you use them) to prevent excessive drop of blood pressure at night.
- **Cool your bedroom.** Keep your bedroom cooler. Heat increases sweating, which dehydrates.
- **Pee before bed.** Void the bladder before going to bed. This will make the night more comfortable and prevent the need for a bathroom visit.
- **Compress veins.** Wear compression socks to bed especially if you have varicose veins. Compression socks prevent blood from pooling in the legs.
- **Use spices.** Add cayenne powder to your socks at night. This trick improves circulation.
- **Consider wet sock therapy.** For long-term improvement of circulation in the legs consider wet socks, grandma-endorsed therapy for poor circulation.

When the urge is strong and you have to go keep these in mind:

- **Go slow.** If you have to go at night, sit down in bed first and then lean forward; stay like that for a minute and only then get up. Slow maneuvering prevents blood pressure from rapidly sinking.
- **Go easy.** Do not strain while on a toilet. Straining activates the vagus nerve. Vagus slows down the heart and slower heart means lower blood pressure.
- **Move your legs first.** Don't jump suddenly out of bed in the morning. Start slow. Rotate your ankles and move your feet up and down. The exercise will activate circulation and push pooled blood up the legs.
- **Sit down when coughing.** Sit down when coughing. Coughing, not unlike straining, slows down the heart rate
- **Sit down when voiding.** Put the shame aside, it is acceptable for males to sit down while peeing.
- **Lean forward.** Hold on to something if you are seeing stars. Immediately bend forward. When you do so blood will shift towards the heart and head giving you some extra time to sit or lie down safely.

Section 3

Things you can test at home

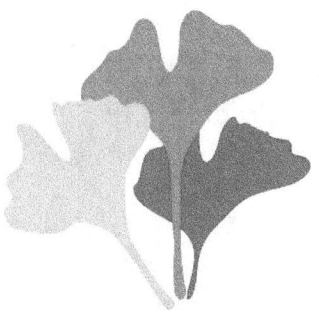

Chapter 11

Ortho... what?

Many things influence morning blood pressure:.night-time dips, cortisol awake effect, hydration, salt intake, alcohol and coffee from the day before. They can have a cumulative effect and add up to a variety of symptoms:

- Sleepiness, fatigue despite sleeping well
- Weakness, faintness even when in bed
- Confusion, light-headedness without any head trauma
- Coldness, chilliness even under covers
- Morning cold, and allergy-like symptoms
- Nausea, lack of appetite

Sluggish morning, sluggish day

For many people morning sluggishness disappears with breakfast, coffee, and moving about. But for some people the standard morning routine may not be sufficient. The yucky feeling and fuzzy head may persist for the entire day getting worse with meals or any sudden movement. Nausea and loss of appetite may show up, but try to not skip meals. It will only make matters worse. Lack of food will lower blood pressure and contribute to body weakness and even bigger brain fog.

This vicious cycle is a common reality for many seniors and people affected by blood pressure irregularities. Unfortunately there is very little a family doctor can do. Surprisingly, you can do much more about it yourself. If fatigue and brain fog persists throughout the day or shows up for no apparent reason it may be due to a frequently hidden underlying condition called orthostatic hypotension.

Ortho... what?

Don`t get scared of that fancy term. Deciphering medical jargon is not difficult. "Orthostatic" translated into plain English means "standing up." "Hypotension" refers to low blood pressure. So "orthostatic hypotension" simply means a drop of blood pressure upon standing up. Since blood pressure drop when standing up is not a healthy response orthostatic hypotension found its way to medical books as a condition describing a cardiovascular anomaly.

Orthostatic hypotension is also called postural hypotension, because it involves changes in the posture. Postural hypotension is very common and causes a big health concern for patients and doctors alike mostly for two reasons:

- Despite its frequency it is seldom recognized
- Despite its frustrating effects there is no easy pharmacological treatment. Only persistent lifestyle adjustments are able to reverse it. *"Health is a Skill, not a Pill."*

Getting to know ortho… what

Have you ever gotten up from sitting to suddenly black out or feel dizzy? Have you ever risen up from bending to see the world spinning? Have you ever lost your balance after climbing a few stairs or doing squats in the gym? If yes, you may have personally experienced episodes of postural hypotension. Postural hypotension, although seldom recognised and diagnosed, causes a real challenge for many people.

Orthostatic hypotension is not a new disease. In fact, it is not a disease at all. It is well known to health practitioners as a nuisance anomaly. But despite its long-standing recognition, the consensus on its clear-cut definition came rather recently in 2011.[38]

Today the name "orthostatic hypotension" does not apply to any minor drop of blood pressure on standing, but has specific diagnostic criteria. The drop needs to be in the magnitude of at least 20 mmHg systolic or 10 mmHg diastolic, rather significant.[39]

Don't get me wrong. Lesser drops of blood pressure do exist and do cause concern. However, from a medical point of view they *cannot be called* orthostatic hypotension. Remember that when you want to discuss this topic with a doctor. A clinician must be very precise when making a diagnosis. If your numbers do not fit perfectly in the criteria you will be pronounced "healthy" even though you are not.

Despite many troubles it causes, orthostatic hypotension is not first on the list to be diagnosed. Very few clinicians routinely test for it and its obscure presentation can elude any patient. Even though blurred vision, recurrent headache, neck ache, palpitations, sweating, nausea, and falls may be obvious and bothersome, not everyone has the foresight to link them to blood pressure. Unpredictability, changeability, and capriciousness of the symptoms complicate the matters for everyone. Some people may have none of the above except for chronic fatigue that comes from nowhere and does not want to go away.[40]

Since orthostatic hypotension is not part of a routine physical, chances are you have never been tested for it. Good news is that the test is simple enough for you to do at home. All you need to have is a blood pressure monitor. Don't skip the test thinking that orthostatic hypotension does not apply to you. Test it and only then you can tell. Studies suggest that even in severe cases 80% of affected may have no apparent symptoms, only long-term side effects.[41]

A hidden epidemic

Postural hypotension is a hidden epidemic. A 2000 study published in *J Hum Hypertens* revealed that half of the adult population suffers sporadic blood pressure drops.[42] The condition increases with age. About 68% institutionalized elderly live with it.[43]

Prescription medications make things worse. Studies show that blood pressure drops affects only one in three elderly that live medication free, but twice that many if they are on meds. Two thirds of seniors who are on three prescription drugs have unstable blood pressure.[44] The incidence goes up with the drug burden. A 2008 study revealed that orthostatic hypotension is present in 35% of seniors who do not take any drugs, 58% in those who take one drug, 60% in those with two, and 65% in those who take three drugs. Medications identified to have the highest orthostatic effect were: Hydrochlorodiazide (65%), Lisinopril (60%), Furosemide (56%), Trazodone (58%), and Terazosin (54%).[45] Check your medicine cabinet.

Orthostatic hypotension seems to also plague people suffering from certain diseases. Half of all people diagnosed with Parkinson`s disease are diagnosed with orthostatic hypotension.[46] Orthostatic hypotension is a frequent feature in diabetics.

Orthostatic hypotension not only causes poorer quality of life, increases life restrictions, but is associated with higher chances of death. Orthostatic hypotension contributes to fainting and falling,[47] and is also linked to heart failure, arrhythmia, and cognitive decline.[48]

Chapter 12

Let's test!

The orthostatic test is simple, but needs to be done properly otherwise errors can obscure the results. You can do the test by yourself, but it would be best if there is somebody with you during the procedure. She/he can help you keep track of time, write down the numbers, and also assist in case you feel dizzy.

How to prepare

1. Ensure your blood pressure monitor is in working order. Check the batteries.
2. Find a sofa/bed/bench you can comfortably lie down on. Keep close to a wall or bench you may hold on to during the test in case you get dizzy.
3. Put the cuff on your left arm and follow the sequence below.

How to test

1. **Lie down**: Stay motionless for about a minute to let blood pressure come down to its resting state.

2. **Test BP**: Start the blood pressure monitor and have somebody record the reading. Have somebody write down all three numbers, including the heart rate. The heart rate number will be useful later

3. **Stand up:** Stand up quickly. Do not sit up, but stand up on both of your feet.

4. **Test BP:** Immediately re-start your blood pressure monitor. Keep your left arm straight. Any bending or arm jerking may invalidate the readings. Have somebody record the results, all three numbers.

5. **Keep standing for three minutes:** Keep on standing motionlessly. If you feel unbearably lightheaded you will need to stop the test and lie down to prevent fainting. Otherwise keep standing for three minutes.

6. **Re-test BP:** Retest your blood pressure at the end of three minutes. Record all three numbers.

7. **10 or more minutes:** If you want to pick up more obscure details keep on standing for another 10 minutes or even longer. Many cases of orthostatic hypotension become evident only after 10 or 20 minutes. Don't talk, watch TV, play games or engage in any mental or physical activity while standing. Any activity may change the reading.

8. **Re-test BP:** Re-test yourself and record all three numbers plus the number of minutes that elapsed from the time you stood up.

What to watch out for?

1. Did your **top** number (systolic) drop by **20 points** from the initial reading at any time during the test?
2. Did your **bottom** number (diastolic) drop by **10 points** from the initial reading at any time during the test?

If you have answered **yes to either one** of these two questions you have experienced orthostatic hypotension.

To ensure that your assessment is reliable repeat the ortho test on different occasions. You can try the test when you feel fatigued, when your blood pressure is low, after a stressful week, on a rainy day, and days when blood pressure is good.

Testing at different times can reveal your individual heart pattern and lets you see whether your body responds to various challenges: weather, stress, fatigue, or hunger. Orthostatic hypotension that happens constantly, regardless of circumstances, is much harder to control and may require medical intervention. Occasional orthostatic events are much easier to deal with and you may be able to control them yourself.

Chapter 13

What does it all mean?

There is a reason why you did the test. First you needed to establish whether your blood pressure behaves normally when you change positions. Secondly, if orthostatic test revealed any imperfections whether you would be able to fix them by yourself.

Here are five possible responses. Only one of them indicates a healthy neurovascular system. The other four reveal cardiovascular flaws. All responses pertain to blood pressure behaviour after standing up.

1. BP **went up**. That`s good. Check chapter 26 for details.
2. BP **went down**, but not low enough for a diagnosis of orthostatic hypotension. Your adrenals may be weak. Read Chapter 27.
3. BP went down enough to recognize **orthostatic hypotension**. Keep on reading and don't skip a page. You will learn a lot from this book.
4. BP **went down after 3 minutes** of standing. You may have delayed orthostatic hypotension. Chapter 14 is for you.

5. BP did not make a large dip, but your **heart started racing**. You may have "orthostatic tachycardia" otherwise called POTS. This condition will be explained in Chapter 15.

Timing makes all the difference

Orthostatic hypotension has three distinctive patterns.[49] The timing of the blood pressure drop makes all the difference to symptoms, causes, and treatments The longer it takes for blood pressure to react the poorer the prognosis.

Less than thirty seconds

Short-lasting blood pressure drops that get caught within 30 seconds are the least concerning. They may lead to temporary dizziness, but rarely to fainting. They are typically "reserved" to younger individuals and do not signify a big health problem. They are also easily rectified, so don't fret too much if you find yourself in this category.

Less than three minutes

Blood pressure dips that are moderately delayed are more concerning and not as innocent. They cause palpitations, hearing and visual disturbances, sweating, or heart pain. The condition is frequently aggravated by diuretics and cardiac drugs, but they are not the only causes. The moderately-delayed orthostatic hypotension may be a sign of a more serious underlying pathology. If you belong to this category you are due for a thorough medical checkup.

More than ten minutes

If a dip in blood pressure does not occur within three minutes, but is extra-delayed, by ten, twenty or maybe even forty-five minutes, the situation is very serious. Delayed orthostatic hypotension tends to occur in very health-compromised individuals and may even signify an autonomic nervous system failure. Watch out for sweating, back pain, and weakness which can appear seconds before a sudden collapse. Older individuals on multiple drugs are the highest risk.

Tips for dealing with orthostatic hypotension

If your test results fall into any of the three orthostatic hypotension scenarios get familiar with the tips below. They will help you avoid sudden dizziness and even prevent falls. They do not repair underlying faulty physiology, but at least they can keep you on your feet and make life more comfortable.

- **Drink water**. Get into a habit of sipping on cold water. That`s especially important if you talk or sweat a lot. Talking and sweating contribute to water loss. Dehydration contributes to fainting; drinking rehydrates and cold water increases blood pressure.[50]
- **Move about**. Moving the legs improves circulation and prevents blood pooling in lower extremities. Whenever possible avoid long car rides as well as prolonged standing. If you are stuck in one place use static exercises to propel blood. You can do them anywhere: on a plane, on a bus or in a waiting room. Contract the muscles below the waist for thirty seconds

at a time. Alternate toe lifting, with bending at the waist, rising legs, or contracting thighs. These exercises will help maintain blood pressure[51] despite many odds.

- **Keep cool**. Heat makes low blood pressure worse. Avoid crowded and heated places. Stay inside air-conditioning malls rather than lying on scorching beaches.

- **Don't panic**. Emotional distress, especially fear is a major contributing factor to fainting.

- **Sit down**. Sit down while yawning, coughing, sneezing, eating, and voiding. These activities can slow down the heart rate, which can be followed by an unexpected blood pressure drop.

- **Avoid blowing**. Sit down while playing a brass instrument. Just like sneezing and yawning, blowing and breath holding slows down heart rate. Even better, switch to playing a piano or a guitar.

- **Stay away from heavy objects**. Be vigilant during and after exercise. Vigorous full body movements are very demanding on the cardiovascular system. Weightlifting is especially challenging. Don't do it unless you are sure of your blood pressure whereabouts.

- **Steady your neck**. Skip neck exercises altogether and leave your neck alone. Certain neck movements and neck rubbing can significantly lower blood pressure.

- **Avoid neck rubs**. Tell your massage therapist about your condition. The neck contains blood pressure regulators and rubbing or massaging them will slow down the heart and produce significant low blood pressure symptoms. Stick to massages below the neck only.

- **Shrink varicose veins**. Take care of those varicose veins. They contribute to blood pooling and prevent blood pressure normalizing surges. Shrink them, or use stockings for a temporary relief.

Keep these simple common sense precautions in mind. Share them with your parents and weaker individuals. Unfit or frail people are most vulnerable to orthostatic hypotension and its consequences.

Chapter 14

An ortho that's late

If your orthostatic test detected a delayed drop of blood pressure this chapter is for you. It will explain the reasons behind erratic blood pressure and why orthostatic delay is of considerable concern.

Is it the nervous system?

Delayed orthostatic hypotension is not to be taken lightly. It should be investigated further because it indicates poor health. This is also the form of orthostatic response that is most easily missed by health care teams. Current clinical setup rarely facilitates testing for a delayed blood pressure drop. The test requires ample space for performing it, a special tilt table, and staff that continuously monitors the patient for thirty to forty-five minutes. Because of these difficulties the test is seldom performed. This leaves an impression that delayed orthostatic hypotension is either unimportant, or constitutes a rare find. Yet despite infrequent diagnosis the problem is not rare at all. A study published in *Neurology* in 2006 found that a delayed blood pressure drop affected 54 % of tested individuals.[52]

Flawless automation is the key to health

The body is armed with multiple mechanisms guarding the stability of blood pressure. Hundreds and thousands of commands are orchestrated in the background without any input of our conscious mind. When performed flawlessly and synced appropriately these automatic processes keep blood pressure at the desired level regardless of exertion, movement, and emotional stress.

When these mechanisms fail, blood pressure fails to respond properly and stays at the mercy of automatic mechanisms coming on or off at unpredictable times. Neuro-hormonal triggers no longer result in action, and stops get ignored when automation malfunctions. Imagine driving a car where neither breaks nor accelerators work when they need to, but activate themselves at random times. When you press a gas pedal the car does not move, but instead headlights flash. When you press a brake pedal at the cross roads your windows open. When you park at a grocery store your car switches parking spots on its own and while driving on a highway it suddenly exits to a side road.

This is exactly what happens with autonomic nervous failure. Body mechanisms turn themselves on at inappropriate times. Timely automation no longer exists. Blood pressure goes down during exercise, and up during sleep. Everything seems to be upside down, unpredictable, and random.

Autonomic nervous system failure is a big problem because all body functions, not only blood pressure, depend on it. Hormone secretion, carbohydrate metabolism, muscular reflexes, respiration, sexual arousal and digestion also rely heavily on the autonomic nervous system. Many of us live with signs of minor auto-malfunctioning without realizing it. Erectile problems, bladder incontinence, erratic handwriting, and bowel irregularity are among them.

Signs of faulty automation

Autonomic failure does not happen overnight. It is a gradual process so elusive that few of us take notice. It is so hidden that even doctors are confused. Signs of automation failure such as erectile difficulties, night-time urination, or fluctuating blood pressure are discussed as if they are separate problems. They are assigned to different specialists who give different treatments for each without factoring in the remaining health issues. Very few clinicians look at the big picture and many falsely believe that above symptoms are inevitable parts of a mid-life crisis.

But once the symptoms are evaluated together they can tell a different health story. The story of progressive nervous system degeneration, not a list of annoying, but isolated, and trivial problems. Only when the bigger issue is realized doctors can prioritize better and improve their treatments. Who cares about a dirty keyboard and a battery failure when the entire computer motherboard is crashing! For the same reason, why limit a treatment to a leaky bladder while the whole body automation is failing?

So how does a malfunctioning automation look like? What are the symptoms? Here is a shortened list of concerns that may surface when the nervous system breaks down. Not everyone will experience all of them or in the same way. Not every symptom listed is unique to the nervous system failure.

Earlier signs my include:

- **Bladder** issues: having to pee at night, involuntary urination, lack of sensation of bladder fullness, stress incontinence (urine leaks on coughing or sneezing), urinary frequency without infection[53]
- **Sexual** issues: erectile troubles, impotence, lack of morning erection (!), difficulty with arousal and achieving orgasm, or untimely ejaculation
- **Bowel** problems: more frequent and less solid stools, chronic explosive diarrhea, uncontrollable gas, or diarrhea at night
- Changes in **sweating**: disappearance of sweating, especially on legs

Later signs may be more obvious and more concerning. Among them are:

- Fainting after exercise
- Repeated light-headedness, weakness and easy fainting
- Increasingly fluctuating blood pressure
- Unsteady gait
- Slurring of speech
- Dimming of vision

Other signs that may be present but are seldom considered:

- Chronic one-sided nasal congestion[54]

- Daily headaches or migraines
- Cravings for sugar and/or salt
- Cardiac arrhythmia
- Different blood pressure readings on either arm

Just don't panic

When I was going through a medical school I had to learn about symptoms and diseases they relate to. The more I knew the more I worried. I had plenty of symptoms and that means I had plenty of diseases. After a few medical books I was sure I was suffering from a whole list of medical problems. I had arthritis and liver failure and a rare virus and a few incurable diseases on top of this. But so did my student colleagues. We all were riddled with multiple diseases. But they weren't real. They were a natural effect of sudden increase in our knowledge.

To prevent yourself from creating imaginary diseases from excess knowledge contact a licensed health care practitioner to discuss the symptoms. Bring orthostatic test results with you to help your doctor assess the situation. You will need a thorough checkup and proper diagnosis.

In the meantime, if your blood pressure is highly unstable adjust medication, hydrate better, and avoid sudden movements. If you suffer from bowel, bladder, or sexual issues pay meticulous attention to personal hygiene and open communication with your partner. Remodel the house or get a walking aid if you have unstable gait or difficulty with mobility.

Once the decline of autonomic nervous system is confirmed you will need to put an effort to stimulate its regeneration. Don't expect that a short-term diet or a pill will do. This will be a longer journey. You will be required to maintain continuous lifestyle effort and check your progress with a knowledgeable physician.

Which doctor would be best to help with health restoration? Look for a board-certified/licensed naturopathic doctor/physician before checking out other professionals. Be aware, though, that different countries, states, and provinces have different laws and regulations. What's an orange in one place may be a plum or a goat in the other. In some places training and requirements for naturopathic doctors are at par or even higher than that of medical doctors. In some other places, though, a naturopathic doctor may mean a weekend-trained practitioner that never saw an anatomy book. Enquire so as not to be disappointed.

Chapter 15

POTS, but not for cooking

POTS is an acronym for Postural Orthostatic Tachycardia Syndrome, a fancy medical name given to a speedy heart rate. POTS is a recent addition to a medical dictionary and describes a condition where the heart accelerates fiercely when a person stands up.

Postural Orthostatic Tachycardia Syndrome applies only to adults. Kids have a much faster heart rate and do not fit in the definition of POTS. You can suspect POTS if the heart rate accelerated more than thirty beats per minute during your orthostatic test.[55] Less than thirty beats is normal and does not indicate any health problem.

Palpitations, fatigue, headaches?

Postural Orthostatic Tachycardia Syndrome is responsible for palpitations, light-headedness, shortness of breath, and weakness. Some people with POTS experience blurry vision and even lose consciousness. POTS is frequent in migraineurs and is known to aggravate the headaches. Forty-eight per cent of people with POTS have fatigue and thirty-two per cent suffer from sleep problems.[56]

POTS can cause an unusual symptom: redness and purplish/blotchy skin on the feet. This is not a cosmetic error. Reddening of the skin is due to blood pooling in the legs. More blood in the legs means less blood for the heart, and that causes heart fluttering and consequently faintness on exertion.

Postural Orthostatic Tachycardia Syndrome is five to ten times more common than orthostatic hypotension.[57] But POTS is not just yet another scary genetic disease to worry about. It is a condition frequently caused by lifestyle factors such as dehydration and physical deconditioning.

Deconditioning

What is deconditioning? You may have guessed that deconditioning is an opposite to conditioning. Here is its more official definition: *"Deconditioning is adaptation of an organism to less demanding environment, or, alternatively, the decrease of physiological adaptation to normal conditions."* What it actually means is that a deconditioned body cannot take challenges because it is less adaptable. Deconditioned body reacts excessively to a small stressor such as a faster stroll or walking upstairs. It is as if the body makes a big deal out of nothing. In people with POTS deconditioning manifests as heart racing upon standing. This "heart panic" is rare in well-conditioned individuals.

Deconditioning is a common occurrence in modern societies. North Americans do not fit into a picture of athleticism. As three quarters are overweight or obese one cannot say we are a population of fitness models. Conveniences, cars, elevators, escalators, scooters, and deliveries do not help with this dilemma. In today's world living is easy. The basics necessities such as transportation, meal preparation, and communication require no physical effort. We no longer need to carry heavy logs, chop wood, and hunt to get a meal. It's enough to click or dial and food magically appears at the door. Saddling a horse or climbing a wagon to enjoy a get together is also a thing of the past. One can see a friend or attend a meeting just by entering a character string with a keyboard. Since there is no longer any need for physical rigor, except finger dexterity, deconditioning is a natural, although not favorable, end-result. Modern conveniences leave many of us physically weakened even in younger years.

Deconditioning is a well-documented phenomenon. It accompanies periods of physical inactivity. It is especially pronounced after a period of bed rest, period of "doing nothing".[58] Bed rest is not always voluntary. It can be a result of illness or accident, but regardless of the reason it always causes substantial changes in body reflexes. During bed rest the heart muscle, just like other muscles, gets weaker. It eagerly adapts to less physically demanding life and shortly follows with diminished effort and weakened pumping.[59]

Bed rest is not different from the chronic chair sitting many of us suffer from. The first one, however, is usually *in*voluntary. It is *caused by* a health problem, whereas the other one is mostly voluntary and *causes* health problems.

A sedentary lifestyle is a well-known, sneaky culprit behind modern deconditioning. It comes on so subtly that many of us have succumbed to it without realizing. How can you check if you have you already fallen victim to it? Here is a quick test: if waking upstairs leaves you huffing and puffing and jogging is out of the question you for sure have.

Once deconditioning sets in it makes all the difference for the immune system. For many chronic fatigue sufferers deconditioning is *the* mysterious factor that prevents recovery. A simple flu that causes bed rest, loss of appetite, and body sweats can turn a deconditioned body into a frail body in an instant. Prolonged illness makes it easy for a deconditioned individual to plunge into a state of chronic fatigue.

People who have low blood pressure and likely also a sedentary lifestyle should consider adding exercise to their daily routine. Strenuous physical exercise, besides improving cardiovascular parameters, can help with resilience. Conditioned individuals recover faster and sometimes that mysterious never-ending post-virus chronic fatigue turns out to be nothing more than an effect of a long-term deconditioning lifestyle.

Need to go physical

You've heard that before. Physical exertion and rigor is a must for maintaining a healthy heart. But for a person with low blood pressure not all exercises are good. If you haven't been moving for a while start with low impact activities like biking, swimming or rowing. Because they are not straining on cardiovascular system they are also safer and more enjoyable.

Avoid jumping, sudden body shifts, and aerobic classes until your heart feels stronger. Excessive cardiovascular stress and quick full-body movements are not for people with hypotension, at least not at the beginning. A process of re-conditioning is an individual journey. If you are lost or not sure how to start seek the assistance of a kinesiologist or a fitness trainer knowledgeable in heart conditions. They will be your best coaches.

Don't avoid exercise because initially it does not feel right or makes you shaky. It is not the exercise that is bad. It is your body that needs to get better. Challenge yourself. Only progressively more difficult activities will bring your body back to strength.

Physical conditioning is the backbone of health. Deconditioning leads to malfunctioning of automatic body reflexes, which direct nervous, immune, digestive, respiratory, endocrine, and circulatory system.[60] This may sound new to you, but physical conditioning is necessary to keep all remote and seemingly unrelated body systems in peak health.

But why should you bother with regular exercise now if you never had before? Why should you waste time on push-ups and squats if strength is not what you care for? Everyone knows that getting into a car, making a phone call, or checking internet does not require any. Although we have gotten convinced that life without exercise is not only possible, but also the less effort the better. Here is the reason why this is not true: continuous poor health is harder than an occasional bout of exercise.

Chapter 16

Keep it at 40 even when older

A blood pressure monitor is indeed a great screening tool. Pulse pressure is another health parameter that can provide valuable information about the body. Pulse pressure is the difference between the top and the bottom number when blood pressure is taken. Pulse pressure can be read from a standard blood pressure monitor without the need for additional equipment. Pulse pressure is calculated from any blood pressure taken at rest, no lying down and standing up is required.

Here is an example of calculation. For blood pressure 120/80 mmHg pulse pressure is 40 (120-80=40). For 159/89 mmHg pulse pressure is 70 (159-89=70). Can you tell what`s pulse pressure for 100/59 mmHg?

A healthy heart will keep pulse pressure at 40. A compromised heart or compromised circulation will drive this number either up or down. The further away from this number pulse pressure is, the bigger the problem. For example, pulse pressure around 50 may be a sign of a minor trouble and pulse pressure of 80 should be seen as a sign of highly increased risk for cardiovascular disease.[61]

When pulse pressure is high

Changes to pulse pressure are very common and they are worth paying attention to. They are usually the first detectable signs of a malfunctioning heart. A wide pulse pressure (above 40) is most commonly caused by stiff arteries. When you see a constantly increased pulse pressure you should check yourself for atherosclerotic plaque.

Healthy arteries are elastic and because of that they accommodate changes in blood flow. Atherosclerotic arteries, arteries that have cholesterol and calcium deposits on their walls cannot do that. They are rigid. They cannot expand. They are narrow and stiff and cannot widen under pressure.

Pulse pressure that consistently reads over 40 should definitely draw your attention. A recent study performed on 8,000 patients revealed that for every ten point pulse pressure increase there is a 20% increase in cardiovascular complications, which includes cardiovascular deaths.[62] This statistics applies also to people whose pulse pressure widened due to medication use.

Arterial deposits cannot be removed with medication. They require major lifestyle changes. Consider making room for unprocessed organic foods, regular exercise, stress reduction, sunshine, and fresh air if you have been diagnosed. In the meantime you can start with supplements. Studies showed that even one pill a day can still make a difference to arterial health.

Folic acid, a popular vitamin, turns out to be a safe and effective method for curbing large pulse pressure. A study published in

American Journal of Clinical Nutrition revealed that even a short-term supplementation of folic acid can produce a visible difference. In that study consumption of 5mg for three weeks resulted in a five point reduction of pulse pressure in a high percentage of individuals.[63] Folic acid does this by reducing arterial deposits and returning arteries to a more elastic state.

Five pressure points may not sound like much, but even this small change is worth aiming for when you consider that wide pulse pressure besides being implicated in heart disease is also linked to strokes[64] and dementia.[65]

When pulse pressure is below 30

If a large pulse pressure is caused by atherosclerosis what's behind a small number? There are two common reasons for it.

Pharmaceuticals. Certain prescription drugs, such as ACE inhibitors, a type of blood pressure medication, can artificially narrow pulse pressure.[66] This may not be good news for people with initially healthy pulse pressure, because the narrower the pulse pressure, the poorer the blood flow.

On the other hand ACE inhibitors can bring a large number back to normal again. But do not jump for excitement though. ACE inhibitors aren't the same as folic acid. They do not lower pulse pressure by cleaning the arteries from cholesterol deposits. ACE inhibitors do not reduce pulse pressure by making arteries more flexible, elastic and youthful, but by cutting off communication between nervous system and blood vessels.

ACE inhibitors are not the only drugs making changes to pulse pressure. Diuretics and other anti-hypertensive pills can do that as well. In fact, any medication may change pulse pressure. If you are on *any* meds your pulse pressure may not reflect your true cardiovascular numbers.

Weak heart pumping. Small pulse pressure may not only come from medication. It can come from a weak heart pumping, which does not mean automatically you have a heart failure. Reduction in heart force can also come from broken nervous system signal or insufficient amount blood arriving at the heart. The latter will be discussed in the chapter about blood loss.

Section 4

Quick and Permanent Fixes

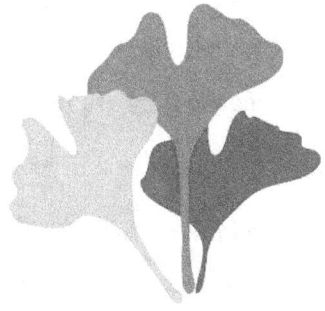

Chapter 17

Blood pressure levelling breakfast

Did you know that, depending on what you eat, breakfasts can lower or increase the heart action? There are many nutritional myths circulating among health enthusiasts. One of them is that banana is good for every heart. People eat bananas because they are rich in potassium and potassium is good for the heart, right?

That wisdom is certainly true in hypertension, but not when one is battling low blood pressure. Bananas and milk won't make mornings more energetic. Foods loaded with potassium and calcium help lower, but not increase cardiovascular numbers. Studies confirmed that the more calcium and potassium in the diet the lower the blood pressure.[67] Should you then stay away from banana pudding entirely? Not at all, but remember to use it at night, when you want to relax, not in the morning, when you need extra energy.

Coffee to the rescue

You may have also fallen for another myth: coffee is bad for you. Before dumping your java entirely consider that coffee can have an extraordinarily energizing effect. This is believed to be at least partially due to coffee's ability to raise blood pressure. Coffee and caffeine's effect on blood pressure has been well researched. Caffeine raises blood pressure. How high depends on the person's cardiovascular health. A study done in 2000 by a University of Oklahoma team found that people with high or normal-high blood pressure have the strongest reaction to caffeine. They respond to it with the highest blood pressure spike.[68] The caffeine effect in people with normal blood pressure is much smaller and also shorter-lasting. Individuals with low or normal blood pressure should not worry about cardiovascular changes due to caffeine. They should enjoy it.

Before adding coffee back to your breakfast, be aware that only real coffee with caffeine is capable of delivering a true cardiovascular boost, so forget about coffee substitutes or decafs. They won't do, regardless of how much you like them and how much you think real coffee is a harmful substance.

Switching to tea?

Did you know that white, green, and black tea comes from the same plant, *camellia sinensis*? Whether white tea becomes green or black is just a matter of timing of harvest and further processing. Green tea turns black after being subject to oxidative fermentation. This process besides changing the color also changes taste, chemical composition, caffeine content and health properties of the leaves.[69]

Seldom anyone hesitates to drink tea due to its bad health effects. Interestingly, a study on green and black tea drinkers has shown that tea, despite having its mild reputation is capable of spiking blood pressure similar to coffee. The spike that comes within thirty minutes after drinking may be substantial. Both green and black tea can cause a spike, but black tea's spike is most intense.

Despite the findings, leave pop alone

Here is another myth: pop increases blood pressure. Pop and energy drinks are frequently used for a pick-me-up effect. Caffeinated varieties will surely produce a wake up effect, but its impact will also depend on another factor: sugar. It turns out, blood pressure effect of pop is not only dependent on caffeine. It also depends on whether soda is sweetened with sugar or artificial sweetener. A ten-week experiment with pop drinkers brought an unusual discovery. Participants who drank sugar sweetened pop saw an increase in blood pressure. In contrast, those who consumed artificially sweetened soda registered lowered numbers at the end of the study.[70]

Despite the above findings I hope that sugar-sweetened pop will be the last thing on your mind when trying to stop the symptoms. Pop regardless of ingredients is a top contributor to ill-health. There is nothing healthy about pop, *especially* if sweetened with artificial sweetener.

Decaf for whom?

Here is yet another myth: decaf is better for you. The need for decaffeination has been debated among people with hypertension, but for people with hypotension decaffeinated beverages should never be recommended.

Unadulterated coffee contains multiple active substances, two of which: caffeine and theobromine are known for cardiovascular effects. Different types of coffee can produce different heart effects due to their different caffeine to theobromine ratio. Decaffeination removes caffeine and leaves theobromine behind. People with low blood pressure should avoid decaf due to its low caffeine high theobromine content.

Theobromine, an alkaloid present in cacao, chocolate, tea, and coffee just like caffeine is capable of altering blood pressure. However, theobromine's action is not the same as caffeine's. Theobromine does not increase blood pressure. It does the opposite: lowers it. Theobromine does that by two actions: widening blood vessels and by diuresis. Because of these two properties: vasodilation and removing excess water, theobromine has been used successfully for lowering blood pressure. Hmmm… wouldn't it only make sense to not use decaf if you have hypotension.

Chapter 18

A pinch about salt

Salt has been deemed as one of the unhealthiest condiments. It has been put next to sugar as another version of a white poison. You were told to stay away from it because it is really bad for you. It can cause high blood pressure, heart failure, hardening or arteries, strokes, and kidney degeneration. Salt is also blamed for causing osteoporosis, blood clumping, cancer of esophagus, and narrowing of arteries.[71, 72]

Health-minded people are quite familiar with the bad side of salt. They put a real effort in reducing its intake. They investigate labels for salt content, stay away from salt-laden junk food, and remove the salt shaker from the table. But despite this enormous health effort they may still end up with some kind of cardiovascular problem.

Overpackaged and oversalted

Salt is a popular food additive and hardly any grocery-store item is void of it. But its wide use is warranted. It is cheap, it delivers flavor and it is a great preservative. It is not surprising that salt can be found everywhere from buns to burgers.

The average American consumes about 2 tsp. of salt a day, equivalent to 3.5g of sodium, double what's recommended. Official guidelines say that one should keep sodium intake somewhere between 1.5 and 2.3 grams a day. Although this is not true for everyone such simplification is necessary to keep the message clear.

Yet despite the message simplicity we keep eating salt "by the bucket". Simply because not everyone studies nutritional information and take out foods seldom come with labels. Even foods that do not taste salty, but sweet, sour, or tart can have a large amount of hidden sodium. The examples may surprise you:

- ½ cup of pasta sauce can contain 0.6g,
- 2 tbsp. of commercial salad dressing 0.4g
- a portion of Eggo waffles 0.6g,
- a portion of Raisin Bran 0.2g,
- 1 cup of vegetable cocktail 0.5g,
- 1 cup of cream-style canned corn 0.7g,
- canned chicken noodle soup 0.8g,
- 1 tbsp. of soya sauce 1g.[73]

There is even salt in colas, fresh buns, and a slice of cheesecake. All processed and ready-made foods contain salt. Consumers that heavily rely on take outs and foods coming in packages end up with unexpected salt-overload. Here is a big surprise: cereals and baked goods are the single largest contributor to dietary sodium intake in US and UK adults.[74] Did you know that?

Are you salt-deprived?

Although statistically we all seem to be overloaded with sodium, many health-conscious individuals end-up being salt-deprived. The reason for it is simple. Healthy people avoid junk and processed foods and a whopping 77% of ingested salt comes from just that.[75] Home-made meals are practically sodium-free.

A risotto made at home has close to zero sodium, but its commercially prepared alternative has over one gram in a portion. Similarly, homemade steak and chips usually end up with less than 0.1 gram, while a standard hamburger and fries has 1.3 grams.[76]

Are you at risk of being sodium deprived? Here are some testing questions to help you with the answer

- Do you eat mostly at home?
- Do you stay away from the salt shaker?
- Do you exercise?
- Are you conscious about drinking plenty of water to hydrate and detoxify?
- Do you talk a lot at work or home?
- Do you sweat when nervous?
- Are you prone to stress and anxiety?

If you answered yes to these questions you may have just discovered the reason behind your low blood pressure: salt insufficiency.

Sodium is not as bad as it is portrayed to be. It is essential for health and we can't live without it. It is also an incredibly important mineral for people with low blood pressure. Sodium is known for its ability to expand fluids, a property you may have noticed yourself. Are you familiar with Chinese restaurant syndrome, when a portion of fried rice and chow mein leave diners thirsty? That's because salt and water go together.

Sodium maintains blood pressure

Our bodies need sodium, and quite a bit of it. Its stores have to be replenished daily as they are easily lost through sweat and urine. Sodium is not just like any other minerals. It does not build bones, help in hormone production or aid in liver detoxification. 85% of all body's sodium is in the blood[77] where it serves an important role. Sodium helps maintain blood pressure.

Since water follows sodium more sodium means more blood volume and that translates to higher blood pressure. More salt in hypertensive individuals can lead to higher blood pressure, but low salt-diet in people with low blood pressure can only deepen hypotension.

This is when a healthy low-sodium diet becomes problematic. It is hard to believe, but one of the most successful treatments for hypotension is regular infusion of intravenous saline solution. A liter of normal saline (water solution containing salt) has been shown to be exceptionally beneficial for people with low blood pressure.[78,79] But don`t google the service yet. There is even a better solution! Instead of finding a doctor that commits to expanding your blood volume weekly, paying money for the service, and wasting an hour sitting in a clinic chair, you may want to dust off your salt shaker instead. It is more convenient and cheaper, does not waste time, and it is definitely tastier than a plastic bag attached to your arm. Getting a salt shaker going in the morning can make a dramatic difference for the rest of the day and lets you think, move, and get your life zest back.

When do I need more salt?

We like routines. They make things predictable, but life is not carved in stone. Don't expect your salt needs to be the same day in, day out. Your salt needs will change with the activity level, weather, and health status. Here are some circumstances that may necessitate more generous sodium intake.

- **Diuretics**: coffee, tea, caffeine drinks, some medication, and weight loss supplements can cause excessive diuresis and subsequent sodium loss
- Diarrhea and **vomiting**: these can cause rapid sodium depletion; watch out especially for vomiting; stomach juices are full of sodium.
- **Heat**: heat causes sweating, sweating depletes sodium; people with low acclimatization have unusually high sodium loss through sweat.[80]
- **Exercise**: intense sweat-producing exercise, especially if done in heat, can cause substantial salt depletion.[81]
- **Physical work**: landscaping, drain digging, construction work can cause obvious sweating, but don't forget that even light gardening in the mid-summer day can do the same.

- **Diet** high in potassium and calcium can cause increased sodium loss through urine.[82] Remember dairy or banana breakfast? Here is another reason why not to.
- **Stress** and anxiety: stress causes sweating of palms, forehead, chest, armpits, or sometimes the entire body; chronic stress can cause massive sodium loss.
- **Infections:** sweating due to infection is not any different than sweating due to exercise, heat or stress; it also causes sodium loss.

Make sure that salt becomes your best friend. Salt helped with my fatigue, so don't be afraid and give it a try. You may be surprised by the results. Here are some quality sources:

- Feta cheese (from organic milk)
- Sauerkraut (naturally fermented)
- Pickles (naturally fermented)
- Roquefort/blue/gorgonzola/camembert cheese
- Parmesan cheese
- Olives
- Bacon (naturally smoked from organic farms)
- Salami (organic)
- Soy sauce
- Salted mackerel, cod

Chapter 19

Do you need more water?

Have you heard the statement that we should drink more water? First, I thought this was a far-fetched oversimplification, but over time I have witnessed how a simple prescription of water made miracles for many patients.

It is true that many of us don't drink the recommended eight glasses a day and despite convenient access to drinking water, we are on the dry side. The elderly are most affected. Heat strokes, confusion, weakness, and heat fainting are common manifestation of dehydration. Although we all know to drink more water there are reasons why we don't.

- We are not very good at distinguishing **hunger** from thirst. And with food tasting better than plain water we end up being overfed and under-hydrated.
- Hydration sensors in the **brain** are not always working. One may not feel thirsty, yet be totally dehydrated.
- Water does not **taste** exciting; pop, beer, coffee chillers, wine are much more palatable. But these are not the same as water. These

are mostly diuretics and will leave negative water balance especially if consumed regularly.

- Drinking water can lead to more frequent **bathroom** visits. These may be inconvenient. No one wants to break a meeting, get off the bus in rush hour, or wake up for the bathroom at the midnight hour, so we drink less to feel more comfortable.

- Leaky incontinent **bladders** are a nuisance. Some people figured that drinking less leads to fewer bladder urges and fewer accidents. Sneezing, coughing, and laughing feel dryer, safer, and more comfortable in a dehydrated state.

- Permanent water **containers** do not fit in small purses and are heavy and one has to keep on carrying it even after use. They can leak making a mess. Lighter one-time use plastic bottles are not environmentally acceptable. Making water conveniently portable requires some thinking.

- Commercial **food** is dehydrating. Common junk snacks such as chips, pretzels, and crackers are dry and salty. So are commercially prepared lunches and dinners.

- We are not good **planners**. We rely on the abundance of coffee and convenience shops and seldom prepare for travel. Few think of taking water in the briefcase or car if fresh drinks are available at any corner. But when faced with lineups, cost, and lack of bathrooms around, we are tempted to suppress the thirst signal.

Do you need more water?

What if you are already good with drinking water? How can you tell if you still need more? Look at your pee. If it looks dark yellow or orange, unless the color is from the meds, you surely need more water. Not sure about the color? Then pinch the skin on the back of your hands and make it stand. If the fold does not flatten in one to three seconds you are dehydrated.

Insufficient hydration commonly causes fatigue, muscle cramps, and headaches. Chronic dehydration leads to constipation, breathing difficulties, stomach ulcers, bladder infections, loss of appetite, insomnia, palpitations, bad breath, brain fog, mood changes, weight gain, and indigestion.[83,84,85] In more serious cases dehydration can even cause seizures, brain swelling, kidney damage, and collapse.[86] Dehydration may lead to low blood pressure.

Ratios matter

Can you be dehydrated even though you drink lots of water and your pee is pale? Surprisingly, you can.

Dehydration is a general term for lack of water. But good hydration does not refer to how much water one drinks, but how much water *remains* in the body. To stay inside the body water needs salt, otherwise it ends up being flushed in the toilet.

Salt and water go together, but not in any random fashion. To work well they must stay in the right proportion. The perfect ratio is 9 part sodium for 1000 parts of water. This is exactly the ratio our blood prefers. Normal saline, an intravenous bag of salty water given in hospitals, which contains exactly 0.9% of sodium, is said to be most hydrating solution available.

Without sufficient salt water cannot stay in tissues. Many concerned folks report that water "goes through them" as soon as it is consumed. It is hard to believe, but despite drinking liters of water one can still stay dehydrated. This is a common paradox in health-conscious individuals.

These are individuals who drink plenty of water, sweat intensely due to exercise, but avoid salt believing it is bad. They never consider that dehydration may the underlying cause behind their low blood pressure, brain fog, fatigue, and poor stamina. They continue to be puzzled as to why, despite putting so much effort into being healthy, they don`t feel good.

Chapter 20

Are you nuts about coconuts?

Coconut water has been used as a standard hydrating beverage in many tropical countries, but its popularity in North America is relatively recent. Coconut water has been marketed, not without reason, as a health-promoting beverage.

Coconut water has significant anti-ageing, anti-carcinogenic, and anti-stroke effects.[87] It is also a powerful antioxidant due to a dense arrangement of inorganic ions. Besides being rich in calcium, magnesium, and sodium it is extremely rich in potassium. Just one cup of coconut water has over 600mg of this mineral,[88] much more than the well-known potassium king, "banana".

Exactly due to its mineral density and a heart-friendly ratio of sodium to potassium coconut water is exceptionally useful for hypotension. Coconut water expands blood volume, which in turn increases blood pressure. One to two cups a day may be enough to put back joy into living.

Coconut water is excellent when one has no access to water, snacks, coffee, or other blood pressure boosters. Coconut water has enough sugars to perk one up, but without giving jitters in return. Ask your doctor first before drinking more than a cup a day. If you have kidney or adrenal problems, diabetic acidosis or heart disease you may be prone to potassium overload and that can cause heart trouble.

It is interesting to note that coconut water is so blood-similar that in case of emergency it could be used directly as a hydrating drip?[89] Filtered coconut water has been used as an intravenous plasma alternative successfully in many countries including Cuba, Honduras, Sri Lanka, Japan, and Solomon Islands.[90] Regardless how exciting it may sound, please refrain from intravenous experimentations. It won't go well. To enjoy coconut water safely limit it to oral intake.

Beware of differences

Before you head out to stack your kitchen pantry with coconut water ensure you are getting the real thing. If you haven't gotten into a habit of reading labels yet, the time is now. Although it may feel tedious, annoying, and bothersome, know that reading labels is as important as reading signs on the road while driving. If you don't you'd end up in trouble.

Don't be tempted to buy any first package that says "coconut water". Read the labels. You may be surprised what's inside and how little of the real thing can actually be there. To avoid disappointment locate the line that says "ingredients" and ensure that it contains only one item: coconut water. If not, put it back on a shelf.

Do not confuse coconut water with coconut milk though. They are two totally different products. The first one is a watery liquid (94% water), the other a white thick substance (only 50% water).[91] Coconut milk won't raise blood pressure. In fact over time it can do the opposite.[92]

Chapter 21

Exercise in the morning? I don't think so!

Is there a special time of the day when you feel your best? Is it right after rising, late afternoon, after coffee or a cold shower?

In people with hypotension energy peaks follow blood pressure peaks. Since blood pressure changes significantly during the day-time hours, change in energy will reflect that. It would be smart to reorganize details of the day to fit biological laws and benefit from lows and highs of the heart.

Mental, physical, and emotional capacity varies throughout the day. Ten a.m. is known as the time of alertness peak.[93] Ten a.m. is the best time for mental activities such as learning, reading, writing, and communicating. At that time you may write your best essay on improving relationships or come up with an innovative solution to world garbage problems, but you most likely won't break the world record in sprint or javelin. Ten a.m. is not the time for performing the most stunning physical feats, especially if your blood pressure keeps low.

We are told that the best time to exercise is in the morning, but what do you do if the body says you are "not up to it?" Should you force yourself into a cardiovascular effort that may not even be paying off? Don't! Listen to your body and shift your fitness routine to p.m. Your body may be much more eager to do physical stunts in the afternoon. Studies showed that the highest cardiovascular efficiency and muscle strength is known to be around 5 p.m. [94] exactly the time when blood pressure is the highest.

Chapter 22

Immune boosting at home

Poor circulation and poor immune system go together. That's why cold feet lead to runny nose, at least in some cases. A combination of low blood pressure and low immune system is extremely common. But to boost the immune system you don't need to give your soul away to the devil, or a Mexican clinic for that matter. You don't need a team of specialist looking over your shoulders twenty-four hours a day, sophisticated hi-tech gadgets, intravenous hookups, or a line-up of newly discovered pharmaceuticals, because the simplest and the most practical method to boost the immune system does not require any of that.

You may also be surprised that you shouldn't be hoping for a referral or any prescription from your medical doctor. Conventional medicine is thin when it comes to building health. Just realize that pharmacy shelves are full of immuno-suppressive drugs, but slim on immuno-boosting pills. Immune system building is not a field conventional medicine excels in, so don't waste your time on standard prescriptions. Science is yet to discover a pill for health, robust circulation, and a strong immune system. Health building is a *skill*, not a capsule or an implant.

Natural medicine is on your side

Natural medicine has more to offer for boosting the immune system. Vitamin C and vitamin D are just two examples. These two vitamins are well-known for their health-promoting properties and have been successfully used even in the most immune-compromised cases, such as cancer or AIDS. The fame of these immune-boosting vitamins has infiltrated conventional medicine over time. Nowadays they are used effectively in the most advanced orthodox clinics. But don't be surprised to find a doctor that got stuck in the past and "doesn't believe in vitamins." They are still around us.

Natural medicine is flourishing. Store shelves are packed with remedies for colds, flus, allergies, fatigue, and poor circulation. Some are worth the money, some aren't worth a glance. But even if you figure out which pills does what, you face yet another problem. The pills continue working only long as you continue taking them. I doubt that being stuck with an ever increasing pill burden is something you aspire to. I suggest a different solution.

Water wonders

If you are not into being chained to the ongoing financial pill drain there is a great immuno-building and blood pressure-regulating solution all in one. It is called hydrotherapy.

Hydrotherapy is an official term for use of water for healing purposes. Water is a foundation of life and is also a prescription for health. Modern hygiene uses water for washing and rinsing to get rid of dirt and germs. But that's only a small fraction of what water can do. From vaginal douches to sitz baths to steam saunas hydrotherapy has wide applications. Water can be used for practically everything from shrinking hemorrhoids to skin rejuvenation. Water can also boost both the immune and cardiovascular system with far better results than pills.

Healing with water is nothing new. The practices were recorded by ancient Egyptians, Romans, Persian, and Greek civilizations.[95] Today hydrotherapy is used by naturopaths, occupational therapists, physiotherapists, and has evolved into sophisticated medical treatments including rehab pools for dogs and cryotherapy in sports medicine. Despite technical advancement and updated scientific insight, water healing properties did not change. Your bathroom shower will work the same way as baths and fountains of the ancient Roman empire pleasing royalties and celebrities.

Immuno-building with water

Immuno-building with water is extremely simple and hugely inexpensive. You do not need any machinery, essential oils, perfumes, lotions, potions, flower petals, or highly advertised and coincidently overpriced health toys. It is such a simple self-care technique that it eliminates the need for big wallets, doctors, nurses, or technicians. Immune and cardiovascular benefits of water are at your fingertips. You can turn your bathroom into a modern health facility even today without paying for costly renovations or specialists.

How does it work then? It starts with your typical shower routine and ends with one-minute immune-building technique. Sixty seconds before ending your shower, turn off hot water. Keep the cold stream running. Stay under the water despite an irresistible urge to run away. This unpleasant moment of sudden chill is necessary. It is not to your detriment. This is exactly when health building happens, so stick with it. Extra sensitive individuals can turn off hot water partially to keep water semi-cold, not chilling-cold. It is a good start, but don't expect it to be as effective as the freezing soak.

Don't cringe! It's worth it!

Studies are very clear that temperature altering hydrotherapy does have an incredible effect on our bodies. Cold invigorates and stimulates. Warmth releases tension and relaxes. Sudden temperature change redirects blood flow, challenges metabolism, and activates detoxification.[96]

A cold shower is not only invigorating, but also changes many vital immune system parameters. Repeated cold water stimulations reduce frequency of infections, increase white blood cell counts, and regulate inflammatory responses. Cold water stress enhances anti-tumor immunity, and boost antiviral and anti-cancer factors.[97] Brief cold hydrotherapy is quickly becoming a novel therapy for weakened and immunocompromised patients, including those with cancer and AIDS.

Cold-water immersion increases metabolic rate and stabilizes core temperature, which is perfect for people with low BBT. Just one hour bath in 20°C (68°F) nearly doubles metabolic rate of the body. Lower temperature boosts it even more. One hour bath at 14°C (57°F) increases the metabolic rate by a whopping 350%! Remember, the colder the water the bigger the boost to body core temperature [98] and that helps with immune system as well as with…. weight loss.

Love your brown fat!

Cold helps build brown fat. Don't panic! Brown fat is not the same jiggly bulge around your navel that you want to get rid of. It is the type of fat you actually want. This type of fat, abundant in newborns, keeps the body temperature up. In adults brown fat gets replaced by less metabolically active and less burnable white adipose tissue, the spare tire you are well familiar with.[99]

Loss of brown fat is not good for the body. Lack of it leads to temperature sensitivity, lower metabolic rate, poorer immunity, and obesity. Studies show that exposure to extreme cold can produce a fifteen-fold increase in brown fat which can result in a nine-pound weight loss over a year.[100] And that's without changing the diet!

Choose your temperature wisely

You have to be patient with brown fat. It does not grow overnight. It takes weeks or months to cultivate it, but don't despair. Hydrotherapy does not only have long-term effects. It can produce significant changes in circulation right away. It can lower or raise blood pressure immediately depending on water temperature. The general rule is: cold water stimulates and hot water inhibits blood flow. To increase heart rate and blood pressure you need a cold bath. A hot bath will slow circulation down and do the opposite.

One hour cold bath at 14°C (57°F) has been shown to cause an 8% increase in blood pressure and a 5% increase in heart rate. To compare, one hour extra warm bath at 32°C (90°F) lowers blood pressure by 12%.[101] Keep that in mind when taking baths. Avoid warm or extra warm baths if you have low blood pressure. Warm water will only contribute to you feeling lethargic and dizzy.

Without showers or baths

Did you know that drinking cold water, not unlike cold baths and showers, also increases blood pressure? Studies show that two glasses of cold water can increase blood pressure by an average 33mmHg systolic and 16 mmHg diastolic points 30 min after ingestion.[102] That effect may be especially observed in older individuals and people with compromised circulation.[103] The same trick can also be used with success by people who get lightheaded after blood donation.

Interestingly, blood pressure rising effect of water is not due to blood volume expansion, but due to stimulation of the nervous system in the same way coffee and cigarettes do. Can a cup of cold water replace espresso while providing the same cardio kick? Apparently yes. Two cups of cold water work the same as two unfiltered cigarettes or 2.5 cups of caffeinated coffee.[104] Amazing!

Chapter 23

Boosting norepinephrine

Hydrotherapy does not fail even when it comes to dealing with the most difficult task: multi-system repair. Studies showed that hydrotherapy can help with hormones, digestion, respiration, bladder control, movement of lymphatics, and many aspects of the immune, circulatory, and nervous systems. Did you know that cold water can reduce edema and muscular pain and a warm compress on the back can double intestinal peristalsis and treat constipation?[105]

Cold water can also provide an aspirin-like effect without side effects of stomach ulcers, aspirin is known-for. Beta-endorphin, a pain reducing neurotransmitter, and cortisol, an anti-inflammatory hormone, can both be boosted by cold showers. Cold water emersions can relieve pain, reduce inflammation, and improve blood flow the same way potent drugs do.

Hydrotherapy effects are extremely powerful. Repeated cold emersions can restore normal function even in difficult to treat chronic fatigue syndrome cases.[106] This is great news, because a pill, whether drug or supplement, for chronic fatigue syndrome is yet to be discovered. How does water do that? Hydrotherapy stimulates hypothalamus-pituitary-adrenal axis, the "mother" of all automation.[107] Cold showers increase production of hormones and neurotransmitters that facilitate it. One of them is norepinephrine, an important blood pressure regulating molecule. People with fatigue and hypotension may be lacking it. An orthostatic test result can tell if norepinephrine production is sufficient. Blood pressure that drops on standing signifies its deficiency.

Norepinephrine is produced "on demand" when blood pressure is challenged by the gravity. When released, norepinephrine, stimulates tiny muscles surrounding arteries. As a result they tighten up, and their increased tension raises blood pressure. When norepinephrine is lacking, tiny muscles do not react and blood pressure fails to go up. Since cold showers stimulate norepinephrine production.[108,109] you have yet another reason to have them.

Chapter 24

Can I take a pill for that?

Before any restorative treatment is effective, one must ensure that the body has all the necessary nutrients for repair. The nervous system just like any other system in the body relies on nutrients that must come from the diet. But eating alone does not guarantee good nourishment. What one eats makes a difference. While processed food is known to be largely devoid of nutrients, homemade meals don't always provide full nutritional insurance. Even *un*processed produce may have inferior nutrient score due to depleted soil it is grown in. Age plays a role as well. It weakens digestion, limits food choices, and lowers nutrient absorption. Add to it diseases of digestive tract, food allergies, cultural and religious restrictions and we have epidemic of malnutrition in a land of plenty.

Blood pressure irregularities and problems with automation are largely aggravated by malnutrition. Nutrient deficiencies not only contribute, but also directly lead to the problem.[110] Vitamin B1, B12, and magnesium are key nutrients, which have to be supplied in sufficient quantities to maintain blood pressure at a healthy level.

Vitamin B1

Deficiency of thiamin (vitamin B1) has been found to be a common cause of nervous system malfunction.[111] A widespread use of high carbohydrate meals and soft drinks seems to be, at least partially, responsible for triggering the problem. High sugar and high carb foods lower blood levels of this vitamin. People with high consumption of sugars are at high risk of developing dysautonomia, which is the basis for erratic blood pressure.[112]

Clinical symptoms of vitamin B1 deficiency, called beriberi, manifest as emotional instability, muscle loss, confusion, tingling in legs and hands, and sometimes swelling of ankles.[113] These symptoms are very common in the elderly. Although a complete depletion of vitamin B1 is rare nowadays, be aware that even a partial depletion can result in inadequate nervous system performance.

Levels of vitamin B1 are tested extremely rarely in clinical settings and you have close to zero chances of being informed about your B1 stores. If your orthostatic test was positive invest in a full spectrum B complex supplement as a precaution. If you are deficient your orthostatic test will improve just in a few weeks.

Vitamin B12

B12 is another B vitamin needed for repair and regeneration of the nervous system. It is essential for heart function, arterial health, and blood flow. B12 is frequently deficient in people suffering from fatigue, anxiety, poor liver detoxification, and heart disease. Vitamin B12 levels, like other nutrients, are also seldom tested. Many people walk about with gross deficiency without realizing it. When patients present with symptoms conventional doctors prescribe heart medication and antidepressants while all they should do is test and prescribe vitamin B12.

There are two main groups most affected by deficiency of B12: people with poor digestion and vegetarians. Poor digestion may manifest as heartburn, indigestion, burping, bloating, and bowel irregularities. Vegetarians may not have such symptoms, because in vegetarians B12 deficiency does not come from lack of absorption, but from dietary insufficiency. Vegetarians may show cardiovascular and nervous system deficiency signs already within a few months after starting B12-deficient diet. Non-cheating vegans will be affected the most, as the plant world is not a good source of B12.

B12 test is a simple blood draw and can be ordered by any licensed doctor. If you decide to skip it, at least consider adding B12 to your supplement regimen as a nutritional insurance. Vitamin B12 is not toxic and if your body does not need it, it will excrete it without any side effects. You may take this vitamin even though your doctor, who performed the test, did not see any deficiency. Your doctor`s diagnosis depends on the lab norms, and these are set to reveal *clinical deficiency*, and not *optimal* body stores. These two are very different.

Normal versus optimal

Twenty-five per cent of American adults have diagnosable *clinical* vitamin B12 deficiency.[114] And according to Statistics Canada over ninety-six per cent of Canadians have "normal" but not optimal numbers.[115]

Optimal range is not set in stone, but every nutritionally oriented doctor can tell you that it is definitely different than the standard lab range. For example, clinical deficiency of vitamin B12 is diagnosed when the levels fall below 148 pmol/L, but optimal levels are three times higher. Suggesting B12 to people with anxiety, toe tingling, fatigue, and forgetfulness seem to produce results even though, according to the lab norms they are absolutely fine. Don't settle for less, because the difference between "normal" and optimal is like surviving versus thriving.

If you decide to take B12 know that not all supplements work. Avoid B12 tablets. They are poorly absorbed. For the same reason don't expect that a multivitamin or a multi B tablet can cover all your B12 needs. Only injections, drops or sublingual tablets/strips that by-pass digestive system can do that. Choose your supplements wisely, and definitely not because they are on sale.

Magnesium

Are you anxious, fatigued, and craving chocolate? Chances are you need magnesium. Magnesium controls nervous system excitability and it is crucial for neurotransmitter production. Modern science strongly links magnesium deficiencies with nervous system disorders, including malfunctioning automation.[116] [117]

Lack of magnesium is a frequent contributor to muscle spasms and twitches, weakness, and bladder incontinence.[118] Confusion, disorientation, and depression can happen even with a small depletion. Magnesium deficiency is common in epilepsy, Alzheimer's, and Parkinson's disease.

Magnesium is found predominantly in dark green leafy vegetables, nuts and seeds, beans and lentils as well as whole grains. But even though your grocery basket can be full of these items you still may end up magnesium deficient. About three quarters of Americans eat magnesium-deficient diet.[119]

Food content of magnesium has drastically declined since 1950. It is not uncommon to see 25%-95% of magnesium reduction in many food sources today.[120] This situation arises mainly for two reasons: processing and soil depletion. Did you know that grains subject to refining lose 80-97% of this mineral? Did you know that collard greens have 84% less magnesium today than three decades ago due to modern soil-depleting agricultural practices?

Our personal dietary preferences can add to the problem. Pop, soda, sweets, and caffeine all leave the body devoid of magnesium.[121] Our unhealthy choices, poor soil quality, and food processing add up. Magnesium deficiency is said to apply to all of us.

*You can find vitamin tests in our **LiveUthing.com** store*

Chapter 25

Turn automatic nutrition on

Good nutrition is a backbone of good health. But how does one ensure good nutrition when soils are depleted, time is scarce, and finances are tight? Aren't conveniences grabbed on the go the best solution for our hurried lifestyles? Fast, tasty and cheap. What else would you ask for? Life is too busy. Why waste time on groceries, meal planning, and cooking.

We are well accustomed to fast take outs and inexpensive deli counters. We got conditioned to consider taste and convenience way before we consider nutrition and health. No one looks up the vitamin score when buying a burger, but everyone is price conscious. Unfortunately, such "value" choices have short legs as poor health gets more expensive over time. Doctors and drugs aren't cheap. Hospital and clinic visits are not really time-savers.

My Provencal soup

Many years spent on investigating nutrition lead me to believe that eating real organic food is an absolute must for good health. Nutritional tests done on my patients were convincing. People who ate organics not only showed more structure-building macronutrients, but also had substantially more micronutrients needed for day-to-day metabolism.

I was born a sceptic, so before knowing this data I was questioning my own organic food choices. Am I jeopardizing my family finances because I buy expensive produce? Would we not be better off eating like everybody else? Should I trade the time spend in the kitchen for lining up in restaurants? Is my family's good health an inevitable consequence of strong genes and not of my culinary effort?

Many people say they cannot afford organics. The "proof" is there. A $4.99 a bunch of raw organic leeks does not stand a chance when compared with $3.99 soup served at a fast food stand. I cannot argue that $3.99 looks more attractive than $4.99, especially when food is ready to eat. So why bother?

I decided to make a true comparison. I pulled out a Provencal vegetable soup recipe from a stash of cookbooks lying around in my library. It needed about nine different ingredients, which I did not have at home. I went grocery shopping and carefully noted the price of each item. When I came back home I put aside the amount of produce needed to make the soup and calculated the price for that amount.

Provencal Vegetable Soup – cost of ingredients

Grocery item	Cost per amount used in soup
Butter, organic	$0.30
Carrots, organic	$0.30
Leeks, organic	$4.00
Celery, organic	$0.30
Thyme, organic	$0.30
White wine, organic	$5.00
Vegetable stock, organic	$2.70
Potatoes, non-organic	$2.70
Beans, canned non-organic	$1.40
Asparagus, fresh non-organic	$3.50
Squash, organic	$6.00
Spinach, organic	$2.50
Peas, frozen non-organic	$0.75
Lemon, organic	$0.50
Total cost (yielded 6 Liters)	**$30.55**
Cost per cup	**$1.27**

Not all items were organic, because my grocery store did not carry those. Despite that my final grocery bill looked for sure larger than a soup for three I could have gotten in my local restaurant. Do I really love cooking that much? I quieted down my doubts and carried on with chopping veggies.

My creation yielded six liters of hardy soup with chunks of vegetables so abundant that they looked as if being squeezed out of the pot. There was no room for floating. The soup was that thick. Yet, this was not a culinary mishap. I like soups that eat like meals. They overshadow highly diluted cheap varieties of fast food slops.

My boys are big eaters, but twenty-four cups of food is not easy to gulp down in one day. The fridge kept the soup for the next three day as we enjoyed it without having to cook again or line up for a nutritionally-impoverished slosh. Real thyme and lemon flavor, at least according to my culinary preference, can never be replaced by artificial seasoning.

My time investment for twenty-four servings of soup was about one and a half hours, which included time for grocery shopping, washing, peeling, as well as cooking. Surprisingly this was less time I would spend driving up to a restaurant, lining up, and waiting to be served ready-to-eat meals for the next three days.

The Provencal soup cost totalled $30.55, which turned out to be $1.27 per serving. I am yet to find a place that serves an organic wine-based soup, not colored water, for less than $1.50.

Cooking at home and even going organics, after a careful analysis, turns out to be tastier, cheaper, and even less time consuming than eating out. I did the math. It is a no brainer. And if you recall from earlier that a vast majority of health problems stem from poor nutrition, it only makes you wonder. Why didn't you start bringing nutrients home earlier? With better nutrition 90% of your health issues would have been taken care of by now.

Section 5

Hidden causes

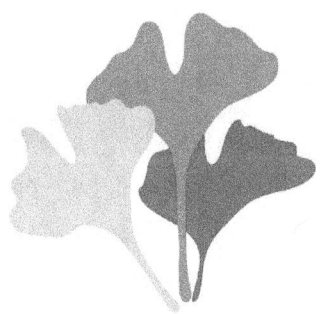

Chapter 26

Blood pressure - your health marker

If you read earlier chapters attentively you know that blood pressure should never just suddenly drop. It is not in its nature. Sudden body movements, jumping, running, or squatting should not make any difference, because autonomic nervous system is supposed to be there to guard the circulation.

Blood pressure drops should be watched carefully, because they mirror autonomic nervous system strength: the bigger the drop the weaker the autonomic self-regulation. Knowing that many functional physicians use orthostatic test to estimate how well the body is doing and how robust it is.

Just as a drop in blood pressure matches poorer health, a sizable increase in blood pressure is a welcomed sign. When the nervous system is fully functional and the circulatory system highly responsive blood pressure spike will be evident and immediate. That's because a healthy body is not only able to compensate for the gravity shift, but also anticipate and prevent any additional circulatory stress.

People with healthy circulation seldom experience dizziness during vigorous exercise sessions, because they can keep blood pressure levelled. People with compromised circulation, on the other hand, get woozy even with minor physical challenges. The difference between the two lies in timing and amount of released norepinephrine. Healthy individuals produce a robust amount of this neurotransmitter. People with low blood pressure don't.

Ortho guide to adrenals

Organs responsible for norepinephrine production are called adrenals. Perfectly working adrenals are capable of levelling blood pressure within a mere few seconds.[122] Speed of their response is crucial. If their response is rapid, no light-headedness is felt even during intense activities. Sluggish adrenals are slower in norepinephrine release and this can be registered as an initial blood pressure drop followed by a delayed blood pressure spike. On the other hand alert and highly responsive adrenals will not only level, but also cause an immediate increase in blood pressure. The healthiest response is said to exist when the top number goes up by 6-10 mmHg points during an orthostatic test [123]. Such a moderate spike is considered an indicator of well-functioning adrenals and a prerequisite for good health. But not all immediate spikes are good. Blood pressure surge of more than 20 points isn't healthy any more.[124]

Find your orthostatic test numbers below to see how your adrenals are doing.

Systolic (top number) behavior on standing	Approximate adrenal function estimation[125]
Increases more than 20 mmHg	Over exaggerated adrenal response
Increases 10-20 mmHg	Strong, but overactive adrenals
Increases 6-10 mmHg	Good adrenal function
Does not change	Fair adrenal function
Drops 1-10 mmHg	Poor adrenal function
Drops more than 10 mmHg	Adrenal exhaustion

Adrenals key to good health

Adrenals are not just any organ. They *are* the soul of life. They not only regulate body automation, but decide on vitality and longevity. Adrenals are so essential to health that even Traditional Chinese Medicine (TCM) recognized their importance many thousand years ago. In TCM adrenals aren't separate organs. They are considered part of the "kidney complex," because they rest on the kidneys and are intimately connected with them.

In TCM, "kidneys" encapsulate the essence of life. When they are weakened, so is life. Hair graying, back pain, ear noises, involuntary ejaculation, leg swelling, fatigue, infertility, poor memory, dizziness, poor eyesight, tooth and bone loss are signs that kidney essence has suffered.

Because TCM falls short in research papers modern medicine has difficult time considering TCM as a compelling source of medical information. Qi, wind, and heat syndromes, that TCM operates on, sound funny and no reputable doctor today would dare to make a wind-liver diagnosis based on a pulse and tongue. It would be laughable and professionally unacceptable.

But these shady ideas that are backed up by zero lab studies turn out not that far-fetched after all. Scientists are only now confirming the roles of adrenals and their key importance in health. So far we discovered that adrenals are involved in blood sugar regulation, lipid metabolism, growth, inflammation, electrolyte balance, sexual response, hormone production, fight and flight and countless other functions. Adrenals are not just limited to norepinephrine production and blood pressure regulation, but orchestrate the entire body.

Modern science is only now catching up to the truths established long before Christ. But even though research keeps on validating eastern concepts we are yet awaiting their full acceptance among western sceptics. It is a slow process. Acupuncture is just one of the examples. Decades of rejections, doubts, objections, discussions, and counterarguments passed before acupuncture was elevated from a useless sham to a medical treatment status. Understandably, due to their narrowly defined paradigm medical researchers had a difficult time comprehending how a seemingly "random" needling of the skin may produce any effect on organs, hormones, or neurotransmitters. It sounded weird that needling a hand would have an effect on the bowels, and needling a foot could change liver function.

The battle to accept acupuncture as a valid therapy is over. But despite its recognition western medical system is still hesitant to embrace eastern concepts that "lack scientific evidence." So far there are no plans to use TCM philosophy as a springboard to accelerate and deepen the understanding of human physiology. Western doctors are too busy prescribing pills and performing surgeries. Energetics is a foreign concept and looks too silly to be bothered with.

But guess what! The ancient wisdom may not have been sucked out of thin air as some people think. With science making progress we are starting to realize that eastern philosophy presents a valuable insight. Not that long ago another discovery was made. The concept that "kidneys" hold the key to long life known to Chinese doctors for thousands of years has specifically been confirmed by modern science just now. This far-fetched idea is no longer a silly absurd, but a scientifically confirmed correlation between adrenal function, health, and longevity. The missing link seems to be a hormone produced by the adrenals, called DHEA.

DHEA is not just any hormone. It is a neurosteroid, a substance that links nervous system to hormones. DHEA is also a grandfather of other hormones. Estrogen, testosterone, cortisol, pregnenolone, and growth hormone all originate from it. These hormones organize body rhythm, its growth, reproduction, activity and rest. When not balanced, hormones produce a whole host of symptoms from hot flushes to insomnia, to obesity to pain. Low DHEA has been linked to inflammation, insulin resistance, poor immunity, infertility, frailty, poor memory, and poor circulation. Low DHEA has also been associated with heart disease, atherosclerosis, osteoporosis, and sexual problems among many others.[126] Several recent studies suggested that DHEA is so vital that it should serve as a marker for longevity.[127,128]

Declining DHEA leads to decline of health, marks the end of robustness and starts the onset of frailness. Weakening of adrenals is echoed by general deterioration, and that includes poorer orthostatic test scores. Orthostatic test should, due to its value, no longer be seen a time-consuming nuisance experiment, but an important marker for general health. Low DHEA, orthostatic failure, and health are correlated. Whether fatigue, burnout, or dysautonomia, "Chinese kidneys" or called by their current name adrenals are always in the picture.

You can find DHEA test in our LiveUthing.com store

Chapter 27

What if you have adrenal fatigue?

Adrenal fatigue is not recognized as a disease by current medical system, so don't expect to get such diagnosis from your traditionally trained medical doctor. Do not expect your doctor to either use the orthostatic test to measure the health your adrenals. He is likely not familiar with the concept.

Adrenal fatigue is difficult to diagnose because it can present itself with a wide range of symptoms. These can mimic variety of diseases and conditions. Among them are:

- Chronic fatigue, poor memory, "senior moments," confusion, low concentration
- Loss of sex drive
- Cravings for salt and sweets, excessive hunger, alcohol intolerance
- Recurrent infections
- Chronic inflammation or pain
- Inability to handle stress

- Low blood pressure, fluctuating blood pressure, dizziness on standing
- Weakness, low body temperature
- Anxiety, nervousness, apprehension, irritability, insomnia
- Dry, thin skin
- Osteoporosis

Adrenal fatigue is extremely common in our fast-paced, highly stressed society. It actually is an epidemic. Daily pressures, business worries, challenging relationships, difficult working conditions all contribute to adrenal stress. Are your adrenals in perfect health? If not, here is a short list of common factors that upset them:

- Chronic inflammation, chronic pain
- Sleep deprivation, shift work, poor sleeping habits
- Ongoing cumulative environmental toxicity
- Chronic illness, chronic allergies, chronic infections
- Overwork, mental and physical strain
- Trauma, injury, surgery, over-exercise
- Hypoglycemia, starvation, irregular timing of meals
- Poor diet, mal-digestion, mal-absorption, nutritional deficiencies
- Frustration, anger, depression, fear, guilt

You can test adrenal burnout and adrenal fatigue, but you need to know that standard blood tests are not useful. To test the adrenal function you must invest in a modern saliva hormone test. This is the only lab method that can detect early adrenal malfunction. Blood work can only detect a complete or near complete adrenal failure, which is a very late finding. Once the saliva test detects a problem you will be on your way to properly treat the underlying cause of low blood pressure – adrenal weakness.

Chapter 28

What if there is not enough blood?

Low blood pressure can also be caused by insufficiency of blood. But anemia does not have to be a result of a blood gushing wound. Low blood production or chronic blood loss can cause the same. Blood loss does not have to be obvious and not always has to produce immediate symptoms.

For women only

Women are accustomed to regular monthly blood loss during their period and seldom think of it as a possible cause of low blood pressure. But blood loss during monthly period is nothing minor. A woman with an average flow loses about three tablespoons of blood during that time. Women with heavier menses can lose over six tablespoons.[129] Even though such amount does not look significant, it still can make a difference to the energy and blood pressure.

Anemia is one of the leading causes for hypotension. About 10% of North Americans are anemic, that's one out of ten.[130] However, women are ten times more prone to anemia than men for the obvious reason –

periods. Only one out of fifty males suffers from iron deficiency anemia, but as many as one out of five women can be affected by it.[131]

Iron pills are not for everyone

Paleness of skin, tongue, or gums can be a giveaway sign of anemia, but unless you are sure about its cause, do not medicate yourself with iron. Before heading to the health food store or a pharmacy ensure that your body actually needs this mineral. There are many different causes of anemia and iron deficiency is only one of them. You need to confirm that iron supplements can correct it, otherwise you will only end up frustrated.

Ask your doctor for blood test called "ferritin." It is a test that measures iron stores in the body. Medicating with iron when iron storage is normal can result in serious health problems. Iron can worsen inflammation and weaken the immune system.[132] It can even damage the liver. For that reason take iron supplements only when ferritin is low.

Think before going in circles

Starting on iron pills with low ferritin is no brainer, but what should you do if your stores stay low despite taking iron supplements? Do you need to continue taking iron if low ferritin and anemia do not want to go away?

Einstein once said "repeating the same thing over and over again and expecting a different result... that's insanity." So, let's apply Einstein's wisdom here: if a month or three on iron did not boost ferritin levels and anemia persists you must change the strategy or you'll be going in circles. Reassess the cause or change the treatment.

Unfortunately, long-term iron supplementation, despite poor results, is a common practice among health practitioners. I am puzzled as to why such routine treatment is so popular. It is not only ineffective, but also carries side effects that range from digestive upset to immune impairment. Continuous loading with iron in hope that one day iron stores somehow change their mind and magically go up is plain absurd.

Look a bit further

If you continue to battle long-term anemia despite taking iron supplements you need to rethink the approach. Maybe iron pills do not get absorbed. Iron requires a well-acidified stomach and the presence of multiple other nutrients to be digested and built into the hemoglobin. Maybe the stomach does not have enough stomach acid or maybe iron assisting nutrients are missing.

But how can you tell where the problem is? Unfortunately, another blood test is not an option. Nutrients assisting with iron absorption not always can be tested with a blood draw. Although vitamin B12 and folic acid check can easily be done, but neither vitamin A, nor copper or phosphorus can be tested accurately in the blood. For a definite answer you need a different test: hair analysis.

Despite what you may think hair analysis is not done by a hair stylist. It needs to be done by an accredited lab and analyzed by a knowledgeable doctor. Hair analysis, in my opinion, is one of the best tools for assessing mineral reserves and their proportions. Hair analysis can show minerals that blood cannot. That includes selenium, sulfur, manganese, magnesium, vanadium, strontium, boron, and chromium. Consider having hair analysis done regardless whether you have anemia or not. You may discover a few unaccounted for nutritional surprises.

Common causes for low iron

Lacking iron-absorption assisting nutrients is not rare. Under-nutrition is very common and it has many underlying reasons. Here are just a few factors that prevent iron stores from increasing.

- Your **diet is iron deficient**. That is especially true in vegetarians and vegans;
  - ➤ **What to do?** Unless you become an omnivore you may need to add iron supplementation to your menu.
- Your **stomach is too alkaline**. Heartburn is a common indicator of low stomach acidity
  - ➤ **What to do?** Lemon juice is a good remedy to restore it. Drink it before meals.
- You are on **medication** that prevent or reduce iron absorption. Acid blockers are common ones; these are typically given for heartburn.
  - ➤ **What to do?** Do not be afraid to question the necessity or appropriateness of your medications; if you find that they are only managing symptoms you may want to switch to therapy that actually builds your health
- Your **diet blocks iron absorption**. Heavy tea and milk use can do that;

- ➢ **What to do?** Reduce tea and dairy products or use them away from main meals.
- You have **chronic bleeding**;
  - ➢ **What to do?** Find the leaks

Where are those leaks?

Finding the source of chronic blood loss is not a difficult task, but first you must be aware of its existence. Chronic bleeding may be hidden and may neither hurt nor be obvious. Yet despite lack of discomfort don't ignore its possibility, because even a loss of few drops a day can turn you into a white ghost over time.

Here are the most common chronic blood loss sources. Best is to ask a health professional to help you rule out of confirm them.

- Bleeding hemorrhoids (an external and internal exam may be needed)
- Fissures and fistulas within digestive system (they may not hurt, only a doctor can tell)
- Nicked colon polyps (you may need colonoscopy)
- Recurrent bladder infections (pee does not have to look pink)
- Micro-bleeding in urine for other reasons e.g. bladder cancer (urine dipstick test can help)
- Spotting between menses (check your panties regularly)
- Bleeding gums (check spit for reddish color)
- Stomach ulcers (they may not hurt if you are on painkillers)
- Daily use of aspirin and other anti-inflammatory drugs that irritate stomach mucosa (a risk factor for everyone)

- Blood thinning medication and supplements that prevent quick clotting (check skin for easy bruising)
- Micro-bleeding in faeces for other reasons such as colon cancer (ask your doctor for occult blood test in stool)

You can find occult blood test in our Live0thing.com store

Chapter 29

Sugar boost, but no cakes!

Have you ever felt hungry to the point of getting a headache or body shakes? If yes, likely your blood sugar was low. Low blood sugar, also called hypoglycemia, is a frequent contributor to hypotension. Hypoglycemia, despite popular belief, is not reserved to diabetics. It is a very common, but highly under-recognized phenomenon in North America affecting at least half of us.

The word "hypoglycemia" is a source of confusion among practitioners, because it means a different thing to traditionally trained medical doctors and emergency personnel, than to a practitioner trained in functional medicine and health restoration.

Hypoglycemia is not the same a hypoglycemia?!

In an emergency ward diagnosis of hypoglycemia is a serious matter. There is no time for errors, arguments, or uncertainty. Hypoglycemia, if not treated immediately, can lead to permanent brain damage, or even death. For emergency personnel hypoglycemia is a lab number. It is an efficient system everyone understands. Blood glucose that falls below 3 mmol/L (54 mg/dl) is a medical emergency. Assigning one clear number to hypoglycemia prevents any confusion and facilitates prompt resuscitation.

But 3 mmol/L (54 mg/dl) is an extremely low number for glucose. This number can be found only in severe cases. Such severe glucose deficiency is easily detected without much testing, because it is typically accompanied by obvious symptoms such as sweating, fainting, and stupor. Seldom anyone with average health gets there. Hypoglycemia of this kind is reserved to diabetics that use aggressive sugar lowering medication, especially insulin.

There is also a different type of hypoglycemia: hypoglycemia that does not require emergency measures or medical attention. This hypoglycemia has much milder symptoms and does not get close to the emergency lab numbers. This type of hypoglycemia is recognized only by holistic and functional doctors, not medical personnel, and it is exactly the most common type of hypoglycemia occurring today. Since medical doctors are not trained to recognize it, it is consistently overlooked. Too bad, because low blood sugar contributes tremendously to low blood pressure, chronic fatigue, and weight problems.

Do not be frustrated if your doctor cannot find a cause behind low blood pressure and chronic fatigue. Medical etiologies are vastly limited to "genes", "viruses", and "accidents". If you suggest hypoglycemia and your blood sugar is above 3 mmol/L (54 mg/dl) your doctor will only be perplexed about why you even bring it up.

Symptoms of low sugar

Do not be afraid to take health into your own hands. Learn how to recognize odd symptoms, trace the causes, and connect the dots. Here is a list of symptoms that can help you detect hypoglycemia. Read it carefully, because an exceptionally large number of people walk about with minor blood sugar irregularities and symptoms of low blood sugar without realizing it. Do not think that blood sugar has nothing to do with you just because you don't have diabetes. If you are overweight or underweight you likely do have blood sugar issues.

- Sugar cravings
- Fatigue, low energy, see-sawing energy during the day
- Light-headedness, feeling of being spaced out
- Insomnia, difficulty falling asleep or staying asleep
- Temper tantrums, anger, easy frustration
- Anxiety, nervousness, irritability
- Hyperactivity, restlessness, impatience
- Cold hands and feet, body coldness
- Recurrent headaches
- Short attention span
- Forgetfulness, brain fog
- Low physical and mental performance

Oops! I have the symptoms!

To confirm the symptoms you could check your blood glucose, but don't be surprised if the numbers are in the "normal" or, to put it more clearly, non-emergency range. If the symptoms can be corrected by eating sugar you are likely hypoglycemic. Do not make the mistake that your blood glucose level has to be in the emergency zone for you to benefit from tuning up the diet. Blood sugar needs to be corrected before you can correct blood pressure. Why? Because it is low blood sugar that leads to low blood pressure, not low blood pressure that causes low blood sugar.

Caveat! Correcting low blood sugar does not mean eating more sugar. Although this may be true in emergency situation, it is not true in chronic low blood sugar cases. Eating sugar to correct mild hypoglycemia will only make matters worse. A permanent correction of low blood sugar requires a smart nutritional strategy, which involves planning well-balanced meals ahead of time, not eating cakes when hunger strikes.

Follow the rules below. They will be of tremendous help if you have low blood sugar, low blood pressure, and weight problems.

- Eat only small meals; snack rather than eat; this will prevent insulin surges that happen after large meals
- Eat frequently, every two to four hours; this will prevent in-between meal sugar dips
- Choose protein, fat and/or fiber rich meals; these keep sugar steady
- Avoid sweet drinks, including any fruit juices; they are very disruptive to blood sugar
- Avoid sugar substitutions; use normal sugar, but limit portions

- Let go of cakes, cookies, and other sugary junk; they are low blood sugar magicians; they can make hypoglycemia appear from nowhere
- Avoid processed foods; they are usually sugary, starchy, and high in glycemic index
- Avoid overcooked foods; they promote sugar fluctuations more than raw or lightly cooked foods
- Sugar-proof your breakfast; over-processed breakfast cereals can easily start your day with a sugar swing; use eggs or cottage cheese instead

To achieve better health, and not just correct symptoms, choose unprocessed organic produce. Organic produce is high in nutrients and low in toxic agrichemical residue. Organic produce is not only healthy for you and your family, but also good for the entire planet.

Avoid processed food and food imitations that disguise themselves as "food" and worse yet "health food". Processed food is less nutritious, causes health problems for individuals, and adds garbage to the earth. Long-term studies invariably show that junk eating known also as a standard North American diet is the primary cause behind the degenerative decay of humans. We need to finally give up the convenient idea that degenerative diseases are "caught," "gotten," "or passed on genetically", and face the reality: we make them ourselves. Degenerative changes simply reflect cumulative effects of our poor lifestyle and nutritional choices. Older people should not grow decrepit. They should grow wiser. Be the change.

Chapter 30

When good food turns bad

Can good, healthy, fresh, whole, unprocessed food, like a fruit or a vegetable cause unhealthy blood pressure changes? Surprisingly yes, but identifying such can be a bit more complicated than just pointing to a potato or asparagus. There isn't any one food that universally changes blood pressure numbers for everyone. Neither is it true that everyone responds to foods by reacting with a blood pressure change. Nonetheless, the possibility that food contributes to high or low blood pressure symptoms exists for everyone and it is definitely worth looking into.

It's not food allergy or food poisoning

When talking about blood pressure altering foods I am not talking about allergies, although severe allergies can cause dramatic blood pressure changes. Everyone knows what food allergies are. One gets hives, diarrhea, or has difficulty breathing. Some people also get skin rashes, cough, or face swelling. Food allergy is obvious, because it occurs shortly after ingestion of an allergen. It is also predictable. One always gives the same symptoms after eating the same allergen.

Food allergies can be tested. It is a series of skin pricks administered by a physician. Each skin prick is done with a different substance and the diagnosis of allergy is made by observation how skin reacts. If skin swells it indicates an allergen. If it doesn`t the food is cleared as non-irritant. The more aggressive the allergen and the more of it the more skin swelling will be seen. The swelling brings fluids to the skin leaving less for the arteries. A dramatic blood pressure drop can be seen during anaphylaxis, a sudden throat closing due to swelling from allergens such as peanuts or shellfish.

I am not talking about food poisoning either, although the aftermath of explosive bathroom mishaps can lower blood pressure. Food poisoning is obvious and does not require diagnostic tests. Symptoms such as runs, belly ache, nausea, cramps, and liquid smelly poop is self-evident. Detecting the source of evil is not difficult. Whoever shared the food shares the symptoms.

It's hidden food sensitivity

Food allergies or food poisoning can produce hypotension for the above noted reasons, either due to fluid shift or fluid loss, but they do not contribute to chronic erratic blood pressure on a day-to-day basis. Allergies and food poisonings are characteristically distinct, but hidden food sensitivities that contribute to circulatory problems, are not.

Many people think that food reactions are limited to upset stomach and skin rashes, but this is not true. Food sensitivities may contribute to or mimic many health predicaments including migraines, recurrent sinusitis, diabetes, and chronic fatigue. This incredibly important notion of food sensitivities disguising themselves as other ailments started with Dr. Coca's discovery.

Many ailments, one cause

Dr. Coca shocked the world by demonstrating that people can be cured of their chronic ailments by eliminating hidden food sensitivities. Dr. Arthur Fernandez Coca (1875-1959) was a keen observer and a diligent clinician. He wasn't just a medical doctor. He was also a professor, an instructor, a researcher, and founder of a prominent medical journal.[133] During his cadence as an editor-in-chief he established high standards that put *The Journal of Immunology* in the ranks of peer-reviewed publications, which continues to be a source of medical discoveries in immunology. He was exceptional.

Dr. Coca discovered that the body reacts to foods and these reactions can have an amazingly profound effect. They can lead to body-wide inflammation, change in hormone production, and alteration of cardiovascular parameters. Dr. Coca demonstrated that food sensitivities are frequent findings in people with chronic unresolved health issues. What was surprising is that people who had food sensitivities never suspected them. Possibly like you.

Dr. Coca managed to reverse many seemingly unrelated ailments by eliminating hidden food sensitivities. Here is a shortened list of health problems reversed by Dr. Coca just by correcting the diet.

- Weight gain, weight loss, weight fluctuations
- Fatigue
- Nervousness, anxiety, depression, irritability

- Dizziness

- Heartburn, indigestion, constipation

- Stomach, intestinal and gallbladder pain

- Colitis, intestinal bleeding, hemorrhoids

- Epilepsy

- Migraines, recurrent headaches

- Nerve pain

- Sinusitis

- Recurrent infections

- Nose bleeds

- Chronic eye inflammation

- Recurrent canker sores

- Diabetes, blood sugar swings

- Hives

- Chest pain, angina, blood pressure fluctuation[134]

Do you have it?

But do you really have food sensitivities and are your health issues really caused by food? Before rushing to suspect food sensitivity behind every ailment you have you need to learn how to test it. Here is a small tip: people with food sensitivities have an accelerated heart rate, a heart rate that is either fast all day long, or switches between normal slow to rapid. These heart rate changes cannot be attributed to any emotional or physical challenge.

If your morning heart rate starts at 68, and somehow after lunch it accelerates to 104 you should get suspicious. Heart rate in a *healthy* person is remarkably stable. It is not affected by emotions, eating or ordinary movement. Heart rate fluctuations bigger than **ten beats per minute** without physical exertion should be investigated for a hidden stressor, which may happen to be just that... hidden food sensitivity.[135]

Before the test

Hidden food sensitivities are easy to test and relatively easy to identify. You don't need any special equipment except for a watch or a stopwatch and the skill to find your pulse. The test is very accurate except when you are on medication. Blood pressure lowering drugs, anti-depressants anti-histamines, or medication for anxiety will for sure slow down the heart rate and render it useless for food sensitivity assessment.

If you don't know your drugs assume all pills interfere with the test regardless of what they are for. In some cases you would be able to temporary suspend your medication. Ask your doctor for permission. If it is not possible to stay medication-free for the time of the test do the test anyhow. If you get some conclusive results, great! Start with those. If you get mixed, inconclusive, or negative results contact a health provider that is familiar with interpretation of the results in challenging situations.

Finding the pulse

If you don't know how to find your pulse you need to learn this skill before testing your food sensitivities. The easiest place to locate a pulsating artery is at the wrist or neck.

The pulse on your wrist can be found just before the bony bump felt in front of your thumb. Using your index and a middle finger press and hold for five to ten seconds. If it pulsates you found it. If it does not, feel around a different spot nearby.

Pulse on the neck can be found just below the jaw angle. Again, find the most likely spot, press lightly and hold for a few seconds. If it pulsates your fingers are in the right place. Many people find the neck pulse to be easier to find than the wrist pulse.

Once you are successful in finding a pulsating artery you will need to get your heart rate. That's super simple. Count the number of beats for sixty seconds. The heart rate is measured in beats per minute and the number you get is exactly that.

Coca test baselines

Now you are ready to establish your baselines. It is important you get them right. Without solid baselines you won't be able to interpret the results. There are two baseline checks in the morning and one before bed.

First baseline

The first baseline is taken upon waking while still lying in bed. Find your pulse and count your heart rate for sixty seconds. Do it before you move, uncover, or talk. Record the number in a log. This is the only time you will be taking heart rate while not-sitting.

Second baseline

Now you can get up and move about, but don't go to the bathroom or eat breakfast yet. You need to record your second baseline before you do any of that. Sit down for a minute or two and take your pulse. Record the reading in the log.

Third baseline

Although for the remainder of the day you will be recording details of your meals as well as associated heart rates you must remember to also test your third baseline at the end of the day. Remember to sit down and relax for a minute or two just before retiring. Record the number, just like you did with the other two, in your log.

These three baselines are meal-independent measurements and they are meant to reflect your resting heart rate. You will need them to judge the amplitude of your daytime heart accelerations.

Food testing details

Food sensitivity testing procedure is not any different than getting the baselines. The only difference between these two is the timing. Each meal requires four separate measurements. These are to be taken before eating, after eating, a half hour after, and eventually another half hour after that.

Stick to meals made of one food at a time. This will make the analysis least complicated and prevent confusion as to which of the ingredients in the dish is responsible for pulse increase. It`s a no brainer. You can get clearer information from eating a carrot alone than eating a carrot cake with seven other ingredients in it.

Here is a template of two logs you will need for your hidden food sensitivity test: three baselines and four food testing times.

Baseline heart rate (HR) numbers:

Day #	Date	HR in bed	HR on waking	HR before bed

Food sensitivity testing

Day #	Time	Food details	HR before	HR right after	HR ½ hr after food	HR 1 hr after food

The analysis

After four days of testing and recording the data you are ready to interpret your results. Suspect food sensitivities if the heart rate

- goes *above eighty-four* beats per minute *or*
- accelerates *more than ten points* after a meal.

If you detected a clear pattern, congratulations! You have found your hidden food allergies. Take the ingredients out of your menu for two weeks and see what difference that makes. You may be amazed how much power you have over your health just by paying attention to your heart.

If the results are unclear, for example you get different readings for the same food, consider other interfering factors such as city smog, toothpaste, off-gassing materials, house dust, or emotional distress. Remember increase in heart rate only means the body encountered a stressor, but which one you have to find out yourself. If you are unsure how to proceed seek help of a health practitioner versed in detection of environmental sensitivities and familiar with Coca test. You may need to google one.

Chapter 31

Blood pressure, a hologram of health

I hope that by now you understand that the blood pressure test is more than just a check for hypotension. A well-behaved steady blood pressure is a great gauge of good health. Perfectly adjustable blood pressure is an indicator of a strong heart muscle, properly functioning nervous system, elastic arteries, robust adrenals as well as agile body reflexes. A blood pressure monitor is one of the greatest health assessment tools every household should have, because blood pressure and heart rate numbers are reliable indicators of whole body functionality. Those who have the most stable cardiovascular system are the same individuals who have the greatest ability to adjust to life circumstances and those who cope with stress, whether emotional or physical, the best. They are most adaptable.

Erratic heart rate and unpredictable blood pressure swings are indicators of poor health. And although age and genetics can play a role, unless one is over eight decades old, circulatory instability is more attributed to cumulative lifestyle errors: poor food quality, chronic stress, environmental pollution, overuse of medication, lack of sufficient exercise, lack of fresh air and sunshine, rather than to an unfortunate ancestry line.

Health is a skill, not a pill

When the body ails we are conditioned to think in terms of pills. And sure, medication is the fastest way to bring temporary relief for a racing heart, high blood pressure, and shortness of breath, but it is not, in any way, the best long-term solution for health improvement. You *cannot* strengthen your heart, bring back elasticity to your arteries, restore adrenals, and revive your nervous system with blood pressure pills.

To have a robust body, that is resistant to weakness and degenerative changes, one needs to have solid "Health Skills". But in today's world full of controversies and erroneous information, building Health Skills is a skill on its own. To make it easier here are some simple guidelines that will get you on the right tract.

- eat more organic vegetables; say no to junk and processed food
- exercise with intent and intensity; put your heart into every move
- enjoy deeper and more harmonious bonds with others: your spouse, kids, co-workers, and other inhabitants of this planet
- don't hold grudges; shake hands with your enemies; move on
- tickle your photo-responsive cells, bask in the morning sun and don't be afraid of natural daylight
- enjoy nature, hike in deep woods, breathe ionized air and rest your eyes on greens

- take off your work boots, high heels, and sandals, touch the earth; it is your home.

Use Health Skills every day and before you know it you will see a more robust, zestful, stronger, happier, and all around better you!

DrD

References

1 Farhan Bangash and Rajiv Agarwal (2009). Masked Hypertension and White-Coat Hypertension in Chronic Kidney Disease: A Meta-analysis *Clin J Am Soc Nephrol. 2009 Mar; 4(3): 656–664.* doi: 10.2215/CJN.05391008 PMCID: PMC2653652 http://www.ncbi.nlm.nih.gov/pmc/articles/PMC2653652/

2 Perlmuter LC1, Sarda G, Casavant V, Mosnaim AD(2013). A review of the etiology, associated comorbidities, and treatment of orthostatic hypotension [Abstract]. *Am J Ther. 2013 May-Jun;20(3):279-91.* doi: 10.1097/MJT.0b013e31828bfb7f. PMID: 23656967 http://www.ncbi.nlm.nih.gov/pubmed/23656967

3 Bjørn Hildrum, Arnstein Mykletun, Eystein Stordal, Ingvar Bjelland, Alv A Dahl, and Jostein Holmen (2007). Association of low blood pressure with anxiety and depression: the Nord-Trøndelag Health Study. *J Epidemiol & Community Health. 2007 Jan; 61(1): 53–58.* doi: 10.1136/jech.2005.044966 PMCID: PMC2465598 http://www.ncbi.nlm.nih.gov/pmc/articles/PMC2465598/

4 Rita Moretti, Paola Torre, Rodolfo M Antonello, Davide Manganaro, Cristina Vilotti, and Gilberto Pizzolato (2008). Risk factors for vascular dementia: Hypotension as a key point. *Vasc Health Risk Manag. 2008 Apr; 4(2): 395–402.* PMCID: PMC2496988 http://www.ncbi.nlm.nih.gov/pmc/articles/PMC2496988/

5 Charlson ME, de Moraes CG, Link A, Wells MT, Harmon G, Peterson JC, Ritch R, Liebmann JM (2014). Nocturnal systemic hypotension increases the risk of glaucoma progression [Abstract]. *Ophthalmology. 2014 Oct;121(10):2004-12.* doi: 10.1016/j.ophtha.2014.04.016. PMID: 24869467 http://www.ncbi.nlm.nih.gov/pubmed/24869467

6 Pirodda A1, Ferri GG, Modugno GC, Gaddi A. (1999). Hypotension and sensorineural hearing loss: a possible correlation [Abstract]. *Acta Otolaryngol 1999;119(7):758-62.* PMID: 10687931 http://www.ncbi.nlm.nih.gov/pubmed/10687931

7 Arai M1, Takada T, Nozue M. (2003). Orthostatic tinnitus: an otological presentation of spontaneous intracranial hypotension [Abstract]. *Auris Nasus Larynx. 2003 Feb;30(1):85-7.* PMID: 12589857 http://www.ncbi.nlm.nih.gov/pubmed/12589857

8 Isildak H, Albayram S, Isildak (2010). Spontaneous intracranial hypotension syndrome accompanied by bilateral hearing loss and venous engorgement in the internal acoustic canal and positional change of audiography [Abstract]. *H.J Craniofac Surg. 2010 Jan;21(1):165-7.* doi: 10.1097/SCS.0b013e3181c50e11 PMID: 20072012 http://www.ncbi.nlm.nih.gov/pubmed/20072012

9 Jean-Louis Vincent and Diego Castanares Zapatero (2008).The role of

hypotension in the development of acute renal failure. *Oxford JournalsMedicine & Health Nephrology Dialysis Transplantation, 24 (2) p. 337-338.* http://ndt.oxfordjournals.org/content/24/2/337.full

[10] Fanaroff AA1, Fanaroff JM.(2006). Short- and long-term consequences of hypotension in ELBW infants [Abstract]. *Semin Perinatol. 2006 Jun;30(3):151-5.* PMID: 16813974 http://www.ncbi.nlm.nih.gov/pubmed/16813974

[11] Robert D Langer, Theodore G Ganiats, Elizabeth Barrett-Connor (1989). Paradoxical survival of elderly men with high blood pressure. *BMJ, 298, p.1356-1357.* http://www.ncbi.nlm.nih.gov/pmc/articles/PMC1836610/pdf/bmj00232-0032.pdf

[12] June Liu (2011). Correlation Among Different Variables and Life Expectancy. *Undergraduate Journal of Mathematical Modeling: One + Two, 3(2) art.2.* http://scholarcommons.usf.edu/cgi/viewcontent.cgi?article=4820&context=ujmm

[13] Michael Schachter (2004). Diurnal Rhythms, the Renin-Angiotensin System and Antihypertensive Therapy. *British Journal of Cardiology, 2004;11(4).* http://www.medscape.com/viewarticle/490535_2

[14] Silva AP1, Moreira C, Bicho M, Paiva T, Clara JG. (2000). Nocturnal sleep quality and circadian blood pressure variation [Abstract]. *Rev Port Cardiol [Abstract]. 2000 Oct;19(10):991-1005.* PMID: 11126112 http://www.ncbi.nlm.nih.gov/pubmed/11126112

[15] Michael Schachter (2004). Diurnal Rhythms, the Renin-Angiotensin System and Antihypertensive Therapy. *British Journal of Cardiology, 2004;11(4).* http://www.medscape.com/viewarticle/490535_2

[16] A.M. Birkenhäger, A.H. van den Meiracker (2007). Causes and consequences of a non-dipping blood pressure profile. *The Netherlands Journal of Medicine, April 2007 64(4) p. 127-131.* http://njmonline.nl/getpdf.php?id=518

[17] Barksdale DJ, Woods-Giscombé C, Logan JG Stress, cortisol, and nighttime blood pressure dipping in nonhypertensive Black American women [Abstract]. *Biol Res Nurs. 2013 Jul;15(3):330-7.* doi: 0.1177/1099800411433291 PMID: 22472903 http://www.ncbi.nlm.nih.gov/pubmed/22472903

[18] Health Stats. 24-hr ABPM Patterns. Retrieved May 22, 2015 from http://www.healthstats.com/index3.php?page=bp-abpm-24hrabpm-pattern

[19] B. Bouhanick, V. Bongard, J. Amar, S. Bousquel, B. Chamontin (2008). Prognostic value of nocturnal blood pressure and reverse-dipping status on the occurrence of cardiovascular events in hypertensive diabetic patients. *Diabetes & Metabolism Dec 2008 34(6) p. 560-567.* doi : 10.1016/j.diabet.2008.05.005 http://www.em-consulte.com/en/article/195988

[20] Fagard RH (2009). Dipping pattern of nocturnal blood pressure in patients with hypertension [Abstract}. *Expert Rev Cardiovasc Ther. 2009 Jun;7(6):599-605.*

doi: 10.1586/erc.09.35. PMID: 19505275
http://www.ncbi.nlm.nih.gov/pubmed/19505275

[21] Fagard RH (2009). Dipping pattern of nocturnal blood pressure in patients with hypertension. *Expert Rev Cardiovasc Ther. 2009 Jun;7(6):599-605.* http://www.medscape.com/viewarticle/705780

[22] Tan Xu MM, Yong-Qing Zhang MBBS andXue-Rui Tan MD (2012). The Dilemma of Nocturnal Blood Pressure. The *Journal of Clinical Hypertension. 14(11), p. 787–791, November 2012.* DOI: 10.1111/jch.12003 http://onlinelibrary.wiley.com/doi/10.1111/jch.12003/full

[23] Kazuomi Kario, Thomas G. Pickering, Takefumi Matsuo, Satoshi Hoshide, Joseph E. Schwartz, Kazuyuki Shimada (2001). Stroke Prognosis and Abnormal Nocturnal Blood Pressure Falls in Older Hypertensives. *Am Heart Assoc, Scientific Contributions, March 21, 2001.* http://hyper.ahajournals.org/content/38/4/852.full

[24] Thomas G. Pickering MD, DPhil (2008). Ambulatory Blood Pressure and Diseases of the Eye: Can Low Nocturnal Blood Pressure Be Harmful? *The Journal of Clinical Hypertension 10(5), p. 411–414, May 2008.* DOI: 10.1111/j.1751-7176.2008.08048.x http://onlinelibrary.wiley.com/doi/10.1111/j.1751-7176.2008.08048.x/full

[25] Lin-Fang Chen, Ju-Chi Liu, Mei-Yeh Wang, Shiow-Li Hwang, Pei-Shan Tsai (2011). Extreme Nocturnal Blood Pressure Dipping is Associated With Increased Arterial Stiffness in Individuals With Components of the Metabolic Syndrome. *Journal of Experimental & Clinical Medicine 3(3) p.132–136 June 2011.* doi:10.1016/j.jecm.2011.04.007 http://www.sciencedirect.com/science/article/pii/S1878331711000635

[26] Kelli Gibson, Robert Lee Page II (2007). What's Up with Morning Blood Pressure? *Pharmacy Times, June 1, 2007.* Retrieved May 24, 2015 from http://www.pharmacytimes.com/p2p/2007-06-6594

[27] K. Alagiakrishnan (2007). Postural and Postprandial Hypotension: Approach to Management. *Geriatrics and Aging. 2007;10(5):298-304.* http://www.medscape.com/viewarticle/559578_5

[28] J. Hope, (2013). 90% of Britons don't know their blood pressure rate - and more than five million are unaware they have potentially fatal condition. Retrieved July 28, 2015 from DailyMail http://www.dailymail.co.uk/news/article-2421435/90-Britons-dont-know-blood-pressure-rate--million-unaware-potentially-fatal-condition.html

[29] M.E.Dallas (2015). Half of People With High BP Don't Know It. Retrieved July 28, 2015 from WebMD. http://www.webmd.com/hypertension-high-blood-pressure/news/20130903/half-of-people-with-high-blood-pressure-dont-know-it

[30] Chapotot F, Gronfier C, Jouny C, Muzet A, Brandenberger G.(1998). Cortisol secretion is related to electroencephalographic alertness in human subjects

during daytime wakefulness [Abstract]. *J Clin Endocrinol Metab. 1998 Dec;83(12):4263-8.* PMID: 9851761
http://www.ncbi.nlm.nih.gov/pubmed/9851761

[31] Cortisol awakening response. Wikipedia. Retrieved May 24, 2015 from
http://en.wikipedia.org/wiki/Cortisol_awakening_response

[32] Kelli Gibson, Robert Lee Page II (2007). What's Up with Morning Blood Pressure? *Pharmacy Times, June 1, 2007.* Retrieved May 24, 2015 from
http://www.pharmacytimes.com/p2p/2007-06-6594

[33] Addison`s disease. Wikipedia. Retrieved May 26, 2015 from
http://en.wikipedia.org/wiki/Addison's_disease

[34] West DJ, Cook CJ, Beaven MC, Kilduff LP (2014). *J Strength Cond Res. 2014 Jun;28(6):1524-8.* The influence of the time of day on core temperature and lower body power output in elite rugby union sevens players. PMID: 24149752
.http://www.ncbi.nlm.nih.gov/pubmed/24149752

[35] Micturition syncope. Wikipedia. Retrieved August 9, 2015 from
https://en.wikipedia.org/wiki/Micturition_syncope

[36] Guidelines for the diagnosis and management of syncope (2009). *European Heart Journal (2009) 30, 2631–2671.* doi:10.1093/eurheartj/ehp298
http://eurheartj.oxfordjournals.org/content/ehj/30/21/2631.full.pdf

[37] European Society of Cardiology (2009). Guidelines for the diagnosis and management of syncope (version 2009). *European Heart Journal. pp 2631-2671* doi:http://dx.doi.org/10.1093/eurheartj/ehp298

[38] Julian M Stewart (2015). Orthostatic Intolerance (Feb, 02, 2015). Retrieved June 28, 2015 from Medscape http://emedicine.medscape.com/article/902155-overview

[39] Lyall A. J. Higginson (2014). Orthostatic Hypotension, Merck Manual, Professional Version. Retrieved June 28, 2015 from
http://www.merckmanuals.com/professional/cardiovascular-disorders/symptoms-of-cardiovascular-disorders/orthostatic-hypotension

[40] Ar Kar Aung, Susan J. Corcoran, Vathy Nagalingam, Eldho Paul, and Harvey H. Newnham (2012). Prevalence, Associations, and Risk Factors for Orthostatic Hypotension in Medical, Surgical, and Trauma Inpatients: An Observational Cohort Study. *Ochsner J. 2012 Spring; 12(1): 35–41.* PMC3307503
http://www.ncbi.nlm.nih.gov/pmc/articles/PMC3307503/

[41] Scott L Mader,, Identification and Management of Orthostatic Hypotension in Older and Medically Complex Patients, *Expert Rev Cardiovasc Ther. 2012;10(3):387-395.* http://www.medscape.com/viewarticle/759996_11

[42] Owens PE, Lyons SP, O'Brien ET (2000), Arterial hypotension: prevalence of low blood pressure in the general population using ambulatory blood pressure monitoring, *J Hum Hypertens. 2000 Apr;14(4):243-7,* PMID: 10805049,
http://www.ncbi.nlm.nih.gov/pubmed/10805049

[43] Juan J. Figueroa, Jeffrey R. Basford, and Philip A. Low (2008). Preventing and

treating orthostatic hypotension: As easy as A, B, C. Cleve *Clin J Med. 2010 May; 77(5): 298–306*. doi: 10.3949/ccjm.77a.09118 PMC2888469 http://www.ncbi.nlm.nih.gov/pmc/articles/PMC2888469/

[44] Low PA (2008). Prevalence of orthostatic hypotension. *Clin Auton Res. 2008 Mar;18 Suppl 1:8-13*. doi: 10.1007/s10286-007-1001-3. PMID: 18368301 http://www.ncbi.nlm.nih.gov/pubmed/18368301

[45] Poon IO, Braun U (2005), High prevalence of orthostatic hypotension and its correlation with potentially causative medications among elderly veterans, *J Clin Pharm Ther. 2005 Apr;30(2):173-8*, PMID: 15811171, http://www.ncbi.nlm.nih.gov/pubmed/15811171

[46] Ibid http://www.ncbi.nlm.nih.gov/pubmed/18368301

[47] Ooi WL1, Hossain M, Lipsitz LA (2000). The association between orthostatic hypotension and recurrent falls in nursing home residents [Abstract]. *Am J Med. 2000 Feb;108(2):106-11*. PMID: 11126303 http://www.ncbi.nlm.nih.gov/pubmed/11126303

[48] Angelousi A1, Girerd N, Benetos A, Frimat L, Gautier S, Weryha G, Boivin JM (2014). Association between orthostatic hypotension and cardiovascular risk, cerebrovascular risk, cognitive decline and falls as well as overall mortality: a systematic review and meta-analysis. *J Hypertens. 2014 Aug;32(8):1562-71; discussion 1571*. doi: 10.1097/HJH.0000000000000235 PMID: 24879490 http://www.ncbi.nlm.nih.gov/pubmed/24879490

[49] European Society of Cardiology (2009). Guidelines for the diagnosis and management of syncope (version 2009). *European Heart Journal. pp 2631-2671* doi:http://dx.doi.org/10.1093/eurheartj/ehp298

[50] Juan J. Figueroa, Jeffrey R. Basford, and Philip A. Low (2008). Preventing and treating orthostatic hypotension: As easy as A, B, C. Cleve *Clin J Med. 2010 May; 77(5): 298–306*. doi: 10.3949/ccjm.77a.09118 PMC2888469 http://www.ncbi.nlm.nih.gov/pmc/articles/PMC2888469/

[51] Ibid http://www.ncbi.nlm.nih.gov/pmc/articles/PMC2888469/

[52] Gibbons CH, Freeman R. (2006). Delayed orthostatic hypotension: a frequent cause of orthostatic intolerance [Abstract]. *Neurology. 2006 Jul 11;67(1):28-32*. PMID: 16832073 http://www.ncbi.nlm.nih.gov/pubmed/16832073

[53] Michael J. Reichgott (1990). Clinical Methods: The History, Physical, and Laboratory Examinations, 3rd edition, Ch 76 Clinical Evidence of Dysautonomia. http://www.ncbi.nlm.nih.gov/books/NBK400/

[54] Lonsdale D, Shamberger RJ, Obrenovich ME. (2011). Exaggerated Autonomic Asymmetry: A Clue to Nutrient Deficiency Dysautonomia. *WebmedCentral Alternative Medicine 2011;2(4):WMC001854* doi: 10.9754/journal.wmc.2011.001854 http://www.webmedcentral.com/article_view/1854

[55] Postural orthostatic tachycardia syndrome, Wikipedia. Retreived June 28, 2015 from

https://en.wikipedia.org/wiki/Postural_orthostatic_tachycardia_syndrome

[56] Ibid https://en.wikipedia.org/wiki/Postural_orthostatic_tachycardia_syndrome

[57] Postural Tachycardia Syndrome (POTS). Retrieved June 28, 2015 from Physiopedia http://www.physio-pedia.com/Postural_Tachycardia_Syndrome_(POTS)

[58] Underlying Causes of Dysautonomia. Retrieved June 28, 2015 from Dysautonomia International http://www.dysautonomiainternational.org/page.php?ID=150

[59] Benjamin D. Levine, Julie H. Zuckerman, James A. Pawelczyk (1997). Cardiac Atrophy After Bed-Rest Deconditioning, A Nonneural Mechanism for Orthostatic Intolerance. *Circulation, Articles 1997, February 11*. Retrieved June 28, 2015 from http://circ.ahajournals.org/content/96/2/517.long

[60] Underlying Causes of Dysautonomia. Retrieved June 28, 2015 from Dysautonomia International http://www.dysautonomiainternational.org/page.php?ID=150

[61] Sheldon G. Sheps, M.D., High Blood Pressure (hypertension). Mayo Clinic, expert answers. Retrieved June 28, 2015 from http://www.mayoclinic.org/diseases-conditions/high-blood-pressure/expert-answers/pulse-pressure/faq-20058189

[62] Pulse Pressure. Wikipedia. Retrieved June 28, 2015 from https://en.wikipedia.org/wiki/Pulse_pressure

[63] Carolyn Williams, Bronwyn A Kingwell, Kevin Burke, Jane McPherson, and Anthony M Dart (2005). Folic acid supplementation for 3 wk reduces pulse pressure and large artery stiffness independent of MTHFR genotype. *Am J Clin Nutr 2005, February 22.* http://ajcn.nutrition.org/content/82/1/26.full

[64] Peter A. van Zwieten (2001). Drug treatment of isolated systolic hypertension. *Nephrol.Dial.Transplant.(2001) 16 (6): 1095-1097.* doi: 10.1093/ndt/16.6.1095 http://ndt.oxfordjournals.org/content/16/6/1095.full

[65] Peters R, Beckett N, Fagard R, Thijs L, Wang JG, Forette F, Pereira L, Fletcher A, Bulpitt C (2013). Increased pulse pressure linked to dementia: further results from the Hypertension in the Very Elderly Trial – HYVET.*J Hypertens. 2013 Sep;31(9):1868-75.* doi: 10.1097/HJH.0b013e3283622cc6. PMID: 23743809 http://www.ncbi.nlm.nih.gov/pubmed/23743809

[66] Pulse Pressure, Wikipedia. Retrieved June 28, 2015 from https://en.wikipedia.org/wiki/Pulse_pressure

[67] Criqui MH, Langer RD, Reed DM (1989). Dietary alcohol, calcium, and potassium. Independent and combined effects on blood pressure [Abstract]. *Circulation. 1989 Sep;80(3):609-14.* PMID: 2766513 http://www.ncbi.nlm.nih.gov/pubmed/2766513

[68] Terry R. Hartley, Bong Hee Sung, Gwendolyn A. Pincomb, Thomas L. Whitsett, Michael F. Wilson, William R. Lovallo (2000). Hypertension Risk Status and Effect of Caffeine on Blood Pressure. *Hypertension, Scientific Contributions, Jan 27, 2000.* http://hyper.ahajournals.org/content/36/1/137.long [Abstract]

http://www.ncbi.nlm.nih.gov/pubmed/10904026

[69] Youngmok Kima, Kevin L. Goodnera, Jong-Dae Parkb, Jeong Choib, Stephen T. Talcott (2011). Changes in antioxidant phytochemicals and volatile composition of Camellia sinensis by oxidation during tea fermentation [Abstract]. *Food Chemistry 129(4), 1331–1342, 15 December 2011.* http://www.sciencedirect.com/science/article/pii/S0308814611007011

[70] Lenny R. Vartanian, PhD, Marlene B. Schwartz, PhD, and Kelly D. Brownell, PhD (2007). Effects of Soft Drink Consumption on Nutrition and Health: A Systematic Review and Meta-Analysis. *Am J Public Health. 2007 April; 97(4): 667–675.* doi: 10.2105/AJPH.2005.083782 PMCID: PMC1829363 http://www.ncbi.nlm.nih.gov/pmc/articles/PMC1829363

[71] H E de Wardener, G A MacGregor (2002). Harmful effects of dietary salt in addition to hypertension. *Journal of Human Hypertension, April 2002, 16(4) pp 213-223* http://www.nature.com/jhh/journal/v16/n4/full/1001374a.html

[72] Stephen Daniells (2010). Salt's harmful effects may extend to artery hardening. *Food navigator 19-Feb-2010.* Retrieved June 2, 2015 from http://www.foodnavigator.com/Science/Salt-s-harmful-effects-may-extend-to-artery-hardening

[73] Salt Shockers Slideshow: High-Sodium Surprises (Feb 4, 2014). Retrieved June 2, 1015 from http://www.webmd.com/diet/ss/slideshow-salt-shockers

[74] Ian J Brown, Ioanna Tzoulaki, Vanessa Candeias and Paul Elliott (2009). Salt intakes around the world: implications for public health. *International Journal of Epidemiology 38(3) pp. 791-813.* http://ije.oxfordjournals.org/content/38/3/791.full

[75] Mara Detsch. 25 Surprisingly Salty Processed Foods. Retrieved June 2, 2015 from http://www.health.com/health/gallery/0,,20365078,00.html

[76] Ian J Brown, Ioanna Tzoulaki, Vanessa Candeias and Paul Elliott (2009). Salt intakes around the world: implications for public health. *International Journal of Epidemiology 38(3) pp. 791-813.* http://ije.oxfordjournals.org/content/38/3/791.full

[77] Sodium (Na) in Blood (September 04, 2012). Retrieved June 9, 2015 from http://www.webmd.com/a-to-z-guides/sodium-na-in-blood

[78] Michelle Robida (2006). No Difference in the Effectiveness of Albumin Versus Normal Saline for the Treatment of Hypotension in Mechanically Ventilated Preterm Infants. Retrieved June 9, 2015 from University of Michigan Department of Pediatrics Evidence-Based Pediatrics Web Site http://www.med.umich.edu/pediatrics/ebm/cats/albumin2.htm

[79] Greg A. Knoll, Jenny A. Grabowski, Geoffrey F. Dervin and Keith O'Rourke (2003). A Randomized, Controlled Trial of Albumin versus Saline for the Treatment of Intradialytic Hypotension. *Journal of the American Society of Nephrology Nov 12, 2003.* http://jasn.asnjournals.org/content/15/2/487.full

[80] Graham P Bates and Veronica S Miller (2008). Sweat rate and sodium loss during

162

work in the heat. *J Occup Med Toxicol. 2008; 3: 4.* doi: 10.1186/1745-6673-3-4 PMCID: PMC2267797

http://www.ncbi.nlm.nih.gov/pmc/articles/PMC2267797/

[81] Graham P Bates and Veronica S Miller (2008). Sweat rate and sodium loss during work in the heat. *J Occup Med Toxicol. 2008; 3: 4.* doi: 10.1186/1745-6673-3-4 PMCID: PMC2267797

http://www.ncbi.nlm.nih.gov/pmc/articles/PMC2267797/

[82] Sodium. Ministry of Health, Nutrient reference values for Australia and News Zealand. Retreived June 9, 2015 from

https://www.nrv.gov.au/nutrients/sodium

[83] Annie B. Bond (2008). 13 Symptoms of Chronic Dehydration (June 7, 2008). Retrieved June 14, 2015 from http://www.care2.com/greenliving/13-symptoms-of-chronic-dehydration.html

[84] Isaac Eliaz (2012). Are You Chronically Dehydrated? (August 1, 2012). Retrieved June 14, 2015 from http://www.rodalenews.com/chronic-dehydration

[85] Dehydration. Wikipedia. Retrieved June 14, 2015 from

http://en.wikipedia.org/wiki/Dehydration

[86] Dehydration. Mayo Clinic, Diseases and Conditions, Complications, (Feb 12, 2014). Retrieved June 16, 2015 from http://www.mayoclinic.org/diseases-conditions/dehydration/basics/complications/con-20030056

[87] Jean W H Yong (2009). The Chemical Composition and Biological Properties of Coconut (Cocos nucifera L.) Water. *Molecules 2009, 14(12), 5144-5164.* doi:10.3390/molecules14125144

[88] Coconut water. Wikipedia. Retrieved June 9, 2015 from

http://en.wikipedia.org/wiki/Coconut_water

[89] Campbell-Falck D, Thomas T, Falck TM, Tutuo N, Clem K (2000). The intravenous use of coconut water [Abstract]. *Am J Emerg Med. 2000 Jan;18(1):108-11.* PMID: 10674546 .http://www.ncbi.nlm.nih.gov/pubmed/10674546

[90] Karl S. Kruszelnicki (2015). Retrieved from ABC Science on July 20, 2015. http://www.abc.net.au/science/articles/2014/12/09/4143229.htm

[91] Jean W H Yong (2009). The Chemical Composition and Biological Properties of Coconut (Cocos nucifera L.) Water. *Molecules 2009, 14(12), 5144-5164.* doi:10.3390/molecules14125144

[92] Njelekela M, Sato T, Nara Y, Miki T, Kuga S, Noguchi T, Kanda T, Yamori M, Ntogwisangu J, Masesa Z, Mashalla Y, Mtabaji J, Yamori Y. (2003) Nutritional variation and cardiovascular risk factors in Tanzania--rural-urban difference [Abstract]. *S Afr Med J. 2003 Apr;93(4):295-9.* PMID: 12806724 http://www.ncbi.nlm.nih.gov/pubmed/12806724

[93] Circadian Rhythm, Wikipedia. Retrieved June 23, 2015 from

https://en.wikipedia.org/wiki/Circadian_rhythm

[94] Ibid https://en.wikipedia.org/wiki/Circadian_rhythm

[95] Hydrotherapy Wikipedia. Retrieved 23 June 2015 from

https://en.wikipedia.org/wiki/Hydrotherapy

[96] Hydrotherapy information (Sep 20, 2008). Natural Therapy Pages. Retrieved June 23, 2015 from http://www.naturaltherapypages.com.au/article/hydrotherapy

[97] A Mooventhan and L Nivethitha (2014). Scientific Evidence-Based Effects of Hydrotherapy on Various Systems of the Body. *N Am J Med Sci. 2014 May; 6(5): 199–209*. doi: 10.4103/1947-2714.132935 PMC4049052 http://www.ncbi.nlm.nih.gov/pmc/articles/PMC4049052/

[98] Ibid http://www.ncbi.nlm.nih.gov/pmc/articles/PMC4049052/

[99] Brown adipose tissue, Wikipedia. Retrieved 23 June 2015 from https://en.wikipedia.org/wiki/Brown_adipose_tissue

[100] Lizette Borreli (June 24, 2014). Benefits of Cold Showers: 7 Reasons Why Taking Cool Showers Is Good For Your Health. Retrieved June 23, 2015 from Medical Daily http://www.medicaldaily.com/benefits-cold-showers-7-reasons-why-taking-cool-showers-good-your-health-289524

[101] A Mooventhan and L Nivethitha (2014). Scientific Evidence-Based Effects of Hydrotherapy on Various Systems of the Body. *N Am J Med Sci. 2014 May; 6(5): 199–209*. doi: 10.4103/1947-2714.132935 PMC4049052 http://www.ncbi.nlm.nih.gov/pmc/articles/PMC4049052/

[102] Jens Jordan, MD; John R. Shannon, MD; Bonnie K. Black, BSN; Yasmine Ali, BS; Mary Farley; Fernando Costa, MD; Andre Diedrich, MD; Rose Marie Robertson, MD; Italo Biaggioni, MD; David Robertson, MD (1999). The Pressor Response to Water Drinking in Humans, A Sympathetic Reflex? *Circulation, Clinical Investigation and Reports, Sept 15, 1999*. Retrieved June 28, 2015 from http://circ.ahajournals.org/content/101/5/504.full

[103] Leigh MacMillan (2010). Plain water has surprising impact on blood pressure Reporter, Vanderbilt University Medical Center's Weekly Newspaper. Retrieved 23 June 2015 from http://www.mc.vanderbilt.edu:8080/reporter/index.html?ID=9047

[104] Ibid http://circ.ahajournals.org/content/101/5/504.full

[105] A Mooventhan and L Nivethitha (2014). Scientific Evidence-Based Effects of Hydrotherapy on Various Systems of the Body. *N Am J Med Sci. 2014 May; 6(5): 199–209*. doi: 10.4103/1947-2714.132935 PMC4049052 http://www.ncbi.nlm.nih.gov/pmc/articles/PMC4049052/

[106] Ibid http://www.ncbi.nlm.nih.gov/pmc/articles/PMC4049052/

[107] Ibid http://www.ncbi.nlm.nih.gov/pmc/articles/PMC4049052/

[108] Ibid http://www.ncbi.nlm.nih.gov/pmc/articles/PMC4049052/

[109] Norephinephrine, Wikipedia. Retrieved June 28, 2015 from https://en.wikipedia.org/wiki/Norepinephrine

[110] Derrick Lonsdale (2009). Dysautonomia, A Heuristic Approach to a Revised Model for Etiology of Disease. *Evid Based Complement Alternat Med. 2009 Mar; 6(1): 3–10*. doi: 10.1093/ecam/nem064 PMC2644268

http://www.ncbi.nlm.nih.gov/pmc/articles/PMC2644268/

[111] Lonsdale D, Shamberger RJ, Obrenovich ME. (2011). Exaggerated Autonomic Asymmetry: A Clue to Nutrient Deficiency Dysautonomia. *WebmedCentral Alternative Medicine 2011;2(4):WMC001854* doi: 10.9754/journal.wmc.2011.001854
http://www.webmedcentral.com/article_view/1854

[112] Ibid http://www.webmedcentral.com/article_view/1854

[113] Beriberi, Wikipedia. Retrieved June 28, 2015 from https://en.wikipedia.org/?title=Beriberi

[114] Mercola (2009). Warning: Potentially Life Threatening Vitamin Deficiency Affects 25% of Adults Retreived June 28, 2015 from http://articles.mercola.com/sites/articles/archive/2009/05/19/warning-potentially-life-threatening-vitamin-deficiency-affects-25-percent-of-adults.aspx

[115] Government of Canada, Statistics Canada. Vitamin B12 status of Canadians, 2009 to 2011. Retrieved June 28, 2015 from http://www.statcan.gc.ca/pub/82-625-x/2012001/article/11731-eng.htm

[116] Langley WF, Mann D (1991). Central nervous system magnesium deficiency. *Arch Intern Med. 1991 Mar;151(3):593-6.* PMID: 2001142
http://www.ncbi.nlm.nih.gov/pubmed/2001142

[117] Leo D. Galland, Sidney M. Baker, Robert K McLellan. Magnesium Deficiency in the Pathogenesis of Mitral Valve Prolapse. Retrieved June 28, 2015 from http://www.mdheal.org/magnesiu.htm

[118] Mark Sircus (2009, December 8). Magnesium in Neurological Diseases and Emotions. Retrieved June 28, 2015 from http://drsircus.com/medicine/magnesium/magnesium-in-neurological-diseases-and-emotions

[119] Enrivomedica. Ancient Minerals,The Bad News about Magnesium Food Sources. Retrieved June 28, 2015 from http://www.ancient-minerals.com/magnesium-sources/dietary/

[120] Ibid http://www.ancient-minerals.com/magnesium-sources/dietary/

[121] Enrivomedica. Ancient Minerals, Need More Magnesium? 10 Signs to Watch For. Retrieved June 28, 2015 from http://www.ancient-minerals.com/magnesium-deficiency/need-more/

[122] Julian M. Stewart, MD, PhD (2013). Common Syndromes of Orthostatic Intolerance. *Pediatrics. 2013 May; 131(5): 968–980.* PMCID: PMC3639459 doi: 10.1542/peds.2012-2610
http://www.ncbi.nlm.nih.gov/pmc/articles/PMC3639459

[123] Dr. Bryan P. Walsh. The Adrenal Glands. Retrieved August 12, 2015 from Precision Nutrition http://www.precisionnutrition.com/what-do-the-adrenal-glands-do

[124] Orthostatic Hypertension, Wikipedia. Retrieved June 28, 2015 from

https://en.wikipedia.org/wiki/Orthostatic_hypertension

[125] Dr. Bryan P. Walsh. The Adrenal Glands. Retrieved August 12, 2015 from Precision Nutrition http://www.precisionnutrition.com/what-do-the-adrenal-glands-do

[126] Traish AM, Kang HP, Saad F, Guay AT (2011). Dehydroepiandrosterone (DHEA)--a precursor steroid or an active hormone in human physiology..*J Sex Med. 2011 Nov;8(11):2960-82*; PMID: 22032408 doi: 10.1111/j.1743-6109.2011.02523.x. http://www.ncbi.nlm.nih.gov/pubmed/22032408

[127] Ferrari E, Cravello L, Falvo F, Barili L, Solerte SB, Fioravanti M, Magri F. (2008). Neuroendocrine features in extreme longevity [Abstract]. *Exp Gerontol. 2008 Feb;43(2):88-94*. PMID: 17764865 http://www.ncbi.nlm.nih.gov/pubmed/17764865

[128] Blevins JK, Coxworth JE, Herndon JG, Hawkes K (2013). Brief communication: Adrenal androgens and aging: Female chimpanzees (Pan troglodytes) compared with women. *Am J Phys Anthropol. 2013 Aug;151(4):643-8*. doi: 10.1002/ajpa.22300. PMID: 23818143 http://www.ncbi.nlm.nih.gov/pubmed/23818143

[129] Heavy Periods (menorrhagia). Retrieved June 28, 2015 from NHS Choices http://www.nhs.uk/conditions/Periods-heavy/Pages/Introduction.aspx

[130] Prevalence and Incidence of Anemia. Right Diagnosis, Retrieved June 28, 2015 from http://www.rightdiagnosis.com/a/anemia/prevalence.htm

[131] S. Killip, J. Bennett, M.D. Chambers (2007). Iron Deficiency Anemia, *Am Fam Physician. 2007 Mar 1;75(5):671-678*; http://www.aafp.org/afp/2007/0301/p671.html

[132] M. Wessling-Resnick Annu (2010).Iron Homeostasis and the Inflammatory Response. *Annu Rev Nutr. 2010 Aug 21; 30: 105–122*. doi: 10.1146/annurev.nutr.012809.104804 PMC3108097 http://www.ncbi.nlm.nih.gov/pmc/articles/PMC3108097/

[133] The American Association of Immunologists. Arthur Fernandez Coca, M.D. (1875–1959) Brief Bio. Retrieved August 17, 2015 from https://www.aai.org/About/History/Notable_Members/The_JI/Coca_Arthur.html

[134] A. F. Coca (1956). The Pulse Test. Retrieved June 30, 2015 from http://www.soilandhealth.org/02/0201hyglibcat/020108.coca.pdf

[135] A. F. Coca (1956). The Pulse Test. Retrieved June 30, 2015 from http://www.soilandhealth.org/02/0201hyglibcat/020108.coca.pdf